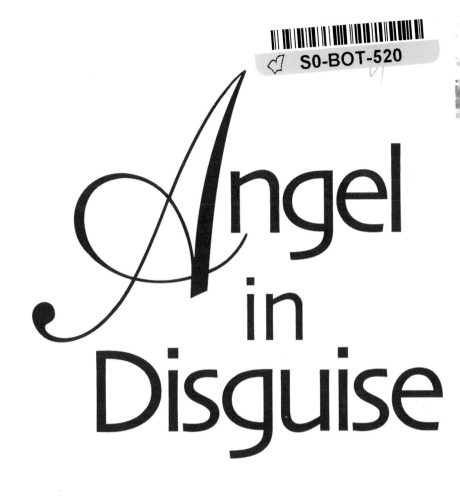

Angel in Disguise

BRIDGING THIS WORLD TO THE OTHER SIDE

by
MarJoe Davidson

ISBN: 1-57901-043-1
Library of Congress Catalog Number: Pending

Cover Design: Michael Lynch
Back cover and inside Photographs: Natalie Wilson

Lesle,

May your life
be fully blessed
from its pages

Marjoe Davidson
6-1-02

MDEES
Box 771 · Concrete, WA 98237
angelcrossing@msn.com
www.mdeespub.com
1-877-699-4229 · 360-873-2305

Contents

ANGEL IN DISGUISE

Introduction

I am MarJoe Davidson and am writing this book as Mary Joe, about the extraordinary life of my mother, Mary Alice Davidson. This vibrant, compelling woman was diagnosed to have lung cancer and twelve tumors on her brain. This book is an account of the final four months that my sisters, brother and I had with this most precious and caring woman that we called 'MOTHER.'

Mary Alice Petray was born in London, Arkansas on August 13, 1912. She was the third born of eight children to Joseph Calvin and Annie Hines Petray. Her father owned a general store and also trapped for furs. Her mother was a housewife and kept quite busy looking after the children. Mother grew up in a loving, close-knit family who took care of each other. It was the time of the Great Depression and all money was needed to keep the family fed, clothed and sheltered. As a teen-ager, Mother worked in the local bakery and would bring home day-old bread for the family. On pay day she would give her paycheck to her mother. To supplement the family's income she also worked in the cotton fields picking cotton, and this paycheck, too, went into the family coffers. Despite her various jobs, Mother continued her schooling while many of her friends had to drop out to help support their families. She had some wonderful memories of those days and shared them with me on many occasions. Mother would get a twinkle in her eyes when she talked about playing basketball for the Malvern High School team. At the time she was five-feet-one inches tall and weighed one hundred pounds. Listening to her reminisce about the games, I could just envision this little ball of pure energy ricocheting around the court.

On August 13, 1936, Mother married James Joseph Davidson, Jr.; it was her twenty-fourth birthday. James was born July 28, 1910 in Russellville, Arkansas. He was the first born of four children to James Joseph and Johnnie Frost Davidson. My mother, Mary Alice, and father, James Joseph had four children: Mary Joe, James David, Patricia Ann and Carol Jean. I was born in Missouri; my brother, James and sister, Patricia were born in Arkansas; and my youngest sister, Carol, was born in Washington State.

In the summer of 1944, my father left Little Rock, Arkansas to work at the Hanford Engineer Works Plant in Washington State. We stayed behind and he sent for us in the fall. Mother, with three children under the age of seven and a fourth child expected in the spring, boarded a train to travel half-way across the United States. It was the height of World War II and the trains were full of soldiers who had returned to the United States from their duty overseas or were going to their next assigned military base. I can remember how helpful and protective several of the soldiers were toward my mother and her little brood. My Dad met us at the train station in Sunnyside, Washington and, as I looked back at the train, some of the soldiers that had traveled the many hundreds of miles with us were standing there smiling. It was if they were saying, "We got your little family to you, James."

Dad had rented a house in Richland for us. Carol Jean was born a few months after we arrived.

As Dad worked for the government, it took care of many of our needs. Our medical, dental and rent costs were very low. Our three bedroom duplex was quite spacious and we had a lot of freedom: we could pick cherries, plums, apples and asparagus on government land. The fruits were amazingly 'Big.' Mother did a lot of canning and baking from the fruits and vegetables that we were able to pick for free. 'FREE'... Little did we know how much that would cost us later in all our lives. The base did have restrictions though; we never saw where Dad worked. He was a civilian employee at Hanford working for the United States government. Dad was very secretive; he never talked about what he did inside the plant. Mother must have sensed the dangers associated with 'The Plant.' She was very insistent that we never go near Dad's lunch pail. I remember it was always kept up out of our reach. As a child I never understood about the lunch pail, but Dad had his reasons and Mother upheld his wishes. Years later, we learned that he worked in the building where the Atomic Bomb was assembled. After the War, Dad became a patrolman guarding the perimeters of the Hanford Plant. It remained off limits to all but those who worked there.

I recall that there were times the town's people were told to stay indoors because the government was spraying for insects. At the time, we didn't question it, but forty years later we found out the spraying was, in reality, radiation being emitted into the atmosphere. The number of total releases from 1943 through 1950 was one hundred and twenty-eight. These releases were equivalent to 530,000 curies of radiation. By way of comparison, at Three Mile Island, the release was 15 curies and the world was concerned! We ate the food and drank the milk and lived our lives not knowing what the United States government, my country, was exposing us to.

We left Richland, Washington in June 1949 and are now beginning to learn of the consequences of having lived there. I received a phone call from Mother sometime in December, 1988. She asked me if I had seen or heard the program on 'Good Morning America' that day. I told her that I hadn't seen the program and why was she wanting to know. She informed me that it had something to do with Hanford, Washington, but that she tuned in to the last of the show so she missed the contents of the program. Mother seemed concerned about what she might have missed but I didn't think at the time that it was something of importance, so I forgot it. Later, I found out that Mother then called Pat to see if she had seen the show. Pat's response was the same as mine. She also called Carol and with that call she found out the terrible news about the releases of radiation on her and her family during the time we lived in Richland, Washington. Carol immediately called the television station to inquire about the program on 'Good Morning America.' The station told her what it was about and gave her a phone number to call in Washington, D.C. for further information. She called and was given a phone number for the Center for Disease Control in Atlanta, Georgia. She made the call and what she found out would change my thinking about this country.

I love my country and would have given my life in defending its boundaries. But now I have these questions: Why did my country do this to me and my family? Why didn't my country love us and the thousands of people in the Hanford area? The United States government let us live there and released radiation on us, then let thousands of people leave the area after the War without telling anyone what they had done.

The information that I received also made me more aware of my own health and left me wondering about the damage the radiation might have had on me. I had two miscarriages during my childbearing years and even my mother and two sisters had miscarriages. Now maybe some questions can be answered. RADIATION . . . What did it do to my body and to the bodies of each member of my family? Why did the government wait to let us know? I found out later that many people who lived in the Hanford area also began asking questions as to why there were more incidents of cancer in people who lived there during the 1940s. The United States government was ordered to open the Hanford files, and we learned our FATE. Now the government is forced to tell the world what they did to their own people!

When we first heard the report about the radiation

releases, Mother's response was, "Why? Oh, why, did they let me keep my little children out there?" That was about all I ever heard my mother say about this devastating news.

Shortly thereafter, my mother, who had never been seriously sick a day in her life, suffered what was diagnosed as a mild stroke. Nine months later, on October 3, 1989, she was diagnosed with cancer.

Mother decided to agree to the treatments prescribed by her physicians. "If there is no change after the chemotherapy and radiation treatments, I will not continue with further treatments," she told her doctors.

The first few treatments of radiation of the head took a toll on her body. She began to refuse to eat. She lost strength in her legs and was unable to walk without the use of a walker or, only, with our help. She needed help taking a bath and getting dressed. After her first infusion of chemotherapy complications arose. She developed pneumonia and became incontinent. She was given insulin due to a chemical imbalance of a hormone.

We respectfully carried out Mother's wishes and eventually brought her to my sister, Carol's, home to live out her last days with dignity. Her loved ones could care for her with help from a local hospice program, and with additional support from the American Cancer Society.

While I'm no expert on death, the hospice program or life after death, I do feel qualified to write about what we experienced. My sisters and I were privileged to witness a remarkable spiritual experience of white light, rays of gold and silver, while

Mother's spirit interacted with each of us for over five and one half hours. This was Mother's last gift to us and it left a impression on me that will last for the rest of my life. This experience validated for me that there is life after death . . . the SPIRIT.

Our experience caring for Mother is also worth sharing because, as the population grows older and health care expenses continue to rise, it is a fact that more Americans will be caring for their loved ones in a home setting, including caring for those who are terminally ill.

The aim of this book is to familiarize those persons who, may one day, become a care giver for a terminally ill person, with how a hospice program works, how to become involved with services that are available, how to interact with family and support personnel, and how my family viewed their part in this incredible transition between life and death.

No words could begin to express the love I hold for my mother and I know my sisters and brother had the same feeling for her. In waiting for death, I want to give an account of feeling and emotions that I, and yes, we, the family had toward this wonderful soul.

Living with death is an everyday process until that person dies. The family has to create as normal a life as possible and yet be available to care for this person.

This was a commitment we made to our dying mother. Her last gift of love to us was filled with many miracles, as we shared a wonderful life after death experience on the Other Side with her. It was after the spiritual experience and the miracle that took place the night before Mother passed on, that we learned we had lived with and in the presence of an angel in disguise.

On January 19, 1990 Mother passed away at the home of my sister with children, granddaughter, great-granddaughter and sister at her side.

This book is a tribute to the memory of Mary Alice Davidson, a remarkable woman in her life-time, and to that Higher Being that we know, without a doubt, allows her to live on

.... IN THE SPIRIT ....

One

Mother was admitted to the hospital on October 3, 1989. Carol had called me at work, "Mary Joe, Mother has just had an x-ray and, Mary, there's a spot . . ." I could not even remember Carol's last words past the word 'SPOT.' I was sick inside; something like that wrong with my mother? Never! Then, as I drifted back, I could hear Carol's voice, "Mary Joe, are you there? Mary . . ."

"Yes, Carol, I'm here. Oh, Carol I can't believe it."

"Neither can I Mary," she sobbed. "The doctor wants to know when Mother last had a chest x-ray. I can't remember."

I could feel the adrenaline begin to flow as I responded, "Carol, Mother had an x-ray when she was in General Hospital* back in December, 1988, when she had her stroke. Call them right now and get those films. They have to release them to you."

Carol answered excitedly, "Mary Joe, that's right. I'll call them right now."

---

* Names of doctors and hospitals have been changed.

She made the call and was told she could pick up the x-rays the next morning.

I arrived at Northwest Medical Hospital* later that afternoon after work. Mother informed me immediately that Dr. Thomas* had called in another doctor, Dr. Jones*, an oncologist, for consultation. Mother had been complaining of dizziness and nausea and now, with a spot on her lung, Dr. Thomas wanted her to have the best medical advice that was available.

More in-depth tests were to be performed the next morning which would entail another scan of the chest and a C.A.T. scan of the head. Since Carol was going to pick up the x-rays the next day from General Hospital, I spent the night with Mother. The x-ray technician arrived early that morning to take Mother for her test.

I sat in Mother's room and waited for Carol to get there . . . I thought back to those words that she had spoken less than twenty-four hours ago; SPOT ON HER LUNGS. These words, and ones I would hear in a few hours, would change my life forever. Carol arrived with a brown folder under her arms, jubilant that she had obtained the all important x-rays. She took the films from their folder.

"Mary Joe, let's take a look at them and see if we can see anything," she said as she put the first x-ray of Mother's lungs against the window, letting the sunlight filter through to give us a clear view. "Do you see anything, Mary Joe?"

"Well I'm no doctor, but I believe that this area looks like a spot or something different." I pointed to the area.

"Mary, I believe you're right."

We then proceeded to look at the other head x-rays; I couldn't see anything in the remaining x-rays but, as I stated, I was no doctor.

"Mary Joe, was Mother nervous when she went down for her test?"

"I think she was, Carol, but you know Mother. We would be the last to know."

We sat together for a while and talked about the discovery that we felt we had made. Our mother had a spot on her lungs in December 1988!! I can't believe that Dr. Matson* had not checked her further, during the nine months that we had her in his office, or had said something during the phone calls that were made about her symptoms and declining condition. I will never understand this doctor's lack of concern and his indifference toward his patient, my mother.

"Mary Joe, let's take the x-rays down to the radiologist."

We had met Dr. Allison* the day before, when she showed us Mother's chest x-ray. We stood at the elevator and we both agreed that we wanted to show Dr. Allison where we thought there was a spot; I suppose to see if we were right.

The elevator door opened and out stepped Dr. Thomas. Excitedly we told him that we had the x-rays from General Hospital and that we were on our way down to give them to Dr. Allison.

He took several steps toward me to be clear of the elevator. "It's worse than we thought," he stated as he looked at me, then at Carol.

'What is this man saying?' I thought. 'What could be worse than a spot on my mother's lungs?'

"Would you rather I tell you both out here or do you want to go to your mother's room and I will tell all of you at the same time."

"Tell us here," we both responded.

Then his words came at me like a knife cutting into my heart and I could feel my legs beginning to buckle under me.

"Your mother not only has a tumor on her lungs, but she has twelve tumors in her head."

This doctor was telling me that the person who I knew as my mother, my traveling companion, my dear friend and often my counselor, had twelve tumors in her head and that by the next day, we would probably know that they were cancerous. I wanted to cry, scream, run as if to leave this terrible news behind me. This couldn't be happening. Mother, mother, my poor mother. Now we must let you know!!

We needed time to get our composure before we went into Mother's room.

As Mother listened to the news, my heart was breaking. I looked at this five-foot-one inch tall, gray-haired woman I had known for fifty-two years, sitting there on the edge of the bed listening to this devastating news. Mother didn't cry, for this was not what she generally did in the presence of her children although I had seen her cry on several occasions. This warm, considerate and loving person, who always thought of her fellow person, was now thinking about her two daughters standing there. She would have to be strong for her daughters. Oh, Mother, Oh, Mother!

The doctor left the room. Mother turned to me and said "Mary, we must call the family."

'Call family,' I thought; 'I can't even talk for fear that I will start crying in front of Mother.'

"Carol get my address book out of my purse," she stated.

So started the calls. First, two calls went out to Pat and James.

"Pat, it's Mary Joe."

"Yes, Mary, I've been waiting to hear from you. I couldn't sleep at all last night. I cried a lot, and I'm still crying off and on. Do you know anything about the C.A.T. scan Mamma had this morning?"

"Yes, Pat, the news is not good."

"Mary Joe, oh god, Mary what do you mean," her voice was breaking and she began to sob.

"Pat, Mother has got . . . " the words were stuck in my throat.

Carol took the phone out of my hand and said, "Pat, Mother has twelve tumors in her head."

Pat became hysterical, crying uncontrollably, but managed to keep talking, "Carol, how is Mamma right now? I, uh, I mean, how did she take the news? Carol, oh Carol, my precious mamma."

Jack, Pat's husband was home, so we felt better knowing that Pat would not be there by herself after we hung up. The next call went to James.

"James, we have the report from this morning's test." I explained to him all that we had been told.

James was silent for a long time. Then he responded, "Uh, uh, uh. Mary Joe tell Mom I'll be over this afternoon." James was not one to say much when around the family. I sometime wondered about this man, my brother, who had in the past been a vice-president for one of the largest trucking companies in the U.S. He is outgoing, aggressive and well liked by all who know him. He progressed from a dock worker, at age eighteen, up to a high management position in the trucking industry . . . but around family, he never talked much.

There were five more calls to make to Pauline, Joan, Aline, Cecil and Junior, Mother's sisters and brothers. Mother talked to each one after we broke the news of her diagnosed cancer. This very strong and independent woman had inherited the MATRIARCH position in the family, passed on by her mother Annie Hines. She was loved and highly respected by all members of her family, who telephoned her frequently. It was as if all would think 'I talked to Mary. She is my rock.'

I took the phone from Mother when she finished talking to Junior. "Junior, it's Mary Joe."

His words were broken and he began to cry. "Mary Joe, I can't believe that this has happened to Mary Alice. I always felt that she would outlive us all."

"I know Junior, I always thought that, too. We're going to be talking to the oncologist, Dr. Jones, later today about the choice of treatments."

"Mary Joe, please keep us informed."

"I will," I said as I hung up the phone.

The family was now aware that we had begun

a journey that would continue to the end of my mother's life.

The nurse came into the room to give Mother a sedative to help her rest through the evening; the doctor felt she would need something after hearing the news. Mother dozed off to sleep.

The phone rang. "Hello," I answered.

"Mary Joe, this is Pat. I called Southwest Airlines and I'm booked to arrive at Dallas Love Field tomorrow night at nine o'clock. Could someone pick me up at the airport? There's no way I can stay down here. I've been crying ever since I hung up the phone talking to you all and to Mamma. I want to be with Mamma; I want to be able to see her and to put my arms around her and to hold her. Mary, I've been praying that she will be okay and that the treatments will help her. Oh, Mary Joe, I don't know what I will do if I lose Mamma."

Tears began to stream down my face as Pat was talking, 'NO TRUER WORDS WERE EVER SPOKEN. WHAT WILL I DO WITHOUT HER?'

Later James arrived at the hospital; Carol and I left the room so James could be alone with Mother. We returned to her room thirty minutes later and as we walked back into the room we could hear Mother telling James, "Don't cry son, everything will work out."

I went over the events of the day and let him know that Pat was due to arrive at the airport the next night and asked him if he could pick her up. He said that there would be no problem meeting Pat as he needed to work late the next day and would be over near Love Field at that time anyway.

Dr. Jones, the oncologist, walked into the room just as Carol and James were getting ready to leave. I was glad that he had caught us all there with Mother, as it gave him an opportunity to tell all of us what he was going to do the next day. The procedure, he explained was a bronchoscopy. He would insert a scope through Mother's mouth into her throat and down into the bronchial tubes to look at and take pictures of the spot that showed up on the chest x-ray. He told her that he wanted her to take the sleeping pill that he had prescribed, as she would need to get a full night's sleep.

He also told her he was starting her on a medication (Decadron) to help reduce pressure in her head due to the tumors located there. I guess that could be the reason that Mother had experienced dizziness all this time. At this time, he said, the medication would be given by intravenous push directly into the veins. Also, since Mother was still nauseated, Phenergan IV was ordered. She would be getting Reglan by intravenous piggyback for her nausea and for reducing any gastric secretions that might cause discomfort.

Dr. Jones left the room. Our conversation was limited to small talk, as I found it hard not to get choked up when I opened up my mouth. James and Carol finally left. I stayed with Mother again that night as I knew that Pat would want to stay with her Thursday night when she arrived from Texas City.

Mother took her sleeping pill and within thirty minutes she had drifted off into a peaceful sleep. I sank back into the comfortable easy chair and cried softly thinking about the day, and before long I was myself free of all that had gone on that day.

Throughout the night I woke up every time Mother turned in the bed . . . just as I remembered doing with my two babies years ago. I was her child and, also, mother to my Mother.

I awoke Thursday around five thirty a.m. and sat crying, holding Mother's hand, and reliving all that had gone on the day before. Suddenly, I felt her hand gently come across the top of my hand.

"Mary Joe, what's wrong?" she said as she moved to a sitting position on the side of the bed.

Before I knew what I was saying I blurted out, "Mother, I'm so angry with you; you led us to believe you would always be okay."

She looked at me with those wonderful caring eyes and responded, "Mary Joe, I'm a human being. I'm just like you. I'm not immortal and I'm so sorry if I've ever led you, any of you, to think that way."

I fell on my knees, to the floor, in front of her and she held my head to her breast and we cried.

ANGEL IN DISGUISE

Two

Mother had talked to several of her friends at the Senior Citizen high-rise where she lived. They received the news with absolute shock and disbelief. Mother was loved by many of the residents that lived there as she had touched many of their lives. "Are you going to return to your apartment, Mary Dee?" was the question that most of them asked after she told them of her disease.

"Sure I am; don't write me off as dead yet," was Mother's reply.

She hung up the phone from her last call, turned to me and looked straight into my eyes and said, "Mary Joe, I believe I will beat this. I will give it my best shot, I know that much."

I remember her words as clear and to the point, but in her eyes the question was there: Mary Joe, will I really make it? I remained silent. My answer was not in words, but my eyes and face must have shown my innermost feelings. 'I hope so, Mother, but the odds are not good. If only it was just the lung cancer, at least you would have a better chance.' Twelve tumors in the brain tips the scales in the other direction.

Dr. Jones sat down with Carol and me and told us the results of the bronchoscopy. The tumor located at the Y of the bronchial tubes was malignant.

The position of the tumor proved to be inoperable. The doctor told Mother the test results and discussed the treatments with her. "I can't promise anything, Mary Alice, but I do know that chemotherapy has proven to be a good treatment when small oak leaf cancer is involved and that is what you have. Also, it is effective when the tumor is rapidly growing, as in your case. The cells are more sensitive to the chemotherapeutic agents when they are undergoing division. This would be my choice of treatment for your lungs, but for the tumors located in the brain, I would recommend radiation treatments."

It was hard to concentrate on what he was saying. Chemotherapy and radiation; these words had been so familiar in my nursing career, but now they were words that seemed so foreign The description of the treatments would be repeated by Dr. Jones once more when all four of Mother's children would be by her side.

The day was a long one, from the time of receiving the news to making the phone calls to family and friends and letting them know the latest findings. Pat would be here today. I knew she would be busy getting her family prepared for her time away from home, so I decided that it would be better to tell her the results of the bronchoscopy when she arrived. Anyway, what could she do except cry and become more upset.

James brought Pat to the hospital where Carol and I met them outside of the emergency room entrance. We all held on to each other and cried for several minutes. I filled Pat in on everything that had transpired that day. As I spoke, the words came between sobs.

"Oh, Mary Joe, I am so mad at that doctor that wouldn't listen to you or Carol."

"I know, Pat," I replied as I thought back to nine months ago when all of this began.

****

I remembered when Mother called my office at two o'clock on December 27, 1988. "Chris, is that you? Can I speak to Mary Joe?"

Chris buzzed me, "Mary Joe it's your mother calling."

"Hi, Mother, how are you doing today?"

"Not so good," was her reply. Then she proceeded to tell me that she had an appointment to see Dr. Waters* the next day. Her voice was weak and her speech slurred. This was not like Mother at all. I talked to her a while longer, and then hung up.

Chris was standing in the doorway. "Mary Joe, what's wrong with Mary? She didn't sound like herself."

"I don't know Chris, but I'm going to call Carol to see if she has talked to Mother today."

Carol picked up the phone on the second ring.

"Carol, Mary Joe here. I just hung up from talking to Mother and she tells me you are taking her to see the doctor tomorrow."

"Yeah, that's right. She's not feeling very peppy."

"Carol, I believe that Mother may be having a stroke or getting ready to have one. Her voice was very slurred and she appeared to be having trouble forming sentences coherently. She may need to see the doctor now or be taken to the hospital emergency room immediately."

"I'll call Mother and Dr. Waters as soon as I hang up," she replied. "I'll call you back as soon as I talk to them, Mary Joe."

It seemed like forever before Carol called me back, but in reality only five minutes had passed by. "Mary Joe, I'm taking Mother to General Hospital Emergency Room. You were right. She doesn't sound like herself. Dr. Waters told me to get her right over to the hospital. Mother says she's not going to go, but I told her I would bring Dwight (Carol's husband) to carry her down the stairs if he had to. She agreed to go when I told her, but she was not very happy that I was making her do this."

"I'll meet you at the hospital, Carol. I'm leaving now."

I was so glad that my friend, Natalie, happened to be at the office. I asked her if she would drive me to the hospital. This was the first of many times that she wound up supporting me and my family through the course of Mother's illness.

Carol was in the waiting room when I arrived. "Mary Joe, Mother is in with Dr. Matson now. I'm so glad that she called you, and that you were able to detect something was wrong."

Mother mentioned that she was dizzy and nauseated. She was admitted into the hospital that evening under the care of Dr. Matson, whom Carol knew.

The next day was the beginning of tests to verify

just what had happened to Mother. I knew without a doubt that it was going to be hard trying to keep her in the hospital for any length of time, as she was never sick and always on the go.

The tests included chest x-rays, a C.A.T. scan of head, carotid scanning, as well as blood work. The results from the chest x-ray and the C.A.T. scan of the head were reported to us by Dr. Matson as being negative; in other words, there was nothing found in these areas.

The doctor stated that the carotid scanning showed build-up of plaque in the veins of the neck. This was probably the cause of her attack. Mother remained in the hospital and after three days she was discharged to go home with medications that Dr. Matson prescribed for her.

Carol usually took Mother back to the doctor's office for her scheduled appointments and would let the doctor know that Mother did not seem to be improving. Dr. Matson, at that point, changed her medication and sent her home to experiment by trying new drugs. Several follow up phone calls were made to Dr. Matson stating that Mother was having problems. Carol had requested, on different occasions, to have some other tests run, but this seemed to fall on the doctor's deaf ears.

Mother, over the next nine months, carried on with her daily routine, but without vim and vigor, as she had in the past.

Mother had an appointment, September 29, to see Dr. Matson and Carol asked me if I could take her, as she was busy that day. I didn't have a class that day at the Nursing School, so I agreed to take

Mother. I was rather glad that I was going because I wanted to talk to the doctor face-to-face. Mother was still complaining of dizziness and nausea during the past nine months, and over a six month period of time, she had lost twenty pounds, going from one hundred and thirty-four pounds to one hundred and fourteen pounds. I was concerned!!

Mother and I arrived at the doctor's office and had to wait only a few minutes. Dr. Matson did a basic examination; blood pressure, temperature, respiration, pulse rate and weight. Mother didn't talk to doctors very much. I guess it was due to the fact that she was never ill. She never developed that bond that comes with a patient/doctor relationship. I explained to the doctor all the symptoms and complaints that Mother was having.

"Dr. Matson, Mother has lost quite a bit of weight and still is nauseated and dizzy. Don't you think that you could put her in the hospital and run some tests to see what is causing this?" I begged.

"NO!! I don't think that would be necessary. I believe that she is experiencing an inner ear infection and that is causing the nausea and dizziness. I'll give you several names of ear doctors. You may choose which one you want to take her to."

"But, Doctor, I think . . . ."

"Look, I'm going to take your mother off all the medication and put her on this one. If, after she sees the ear specialist, she is not any better, we will take it from there."

I took Mother home and went over to the pharmacy to have the prescription filled. I made sure that Mother knew the directions for taking the new medication. I gave her one pill then I headed home.

Shortly after I got home, the phone rang. "Hello."

"Hi, Mary Joe, this is Carol. What did the doctor say about Momma?"

It had been less than an hour since I left Mother and I figured that Carol would have called Mother to find out the report, but I guess she wanted to hear it from me first. I proceeded to give Carol the scoop on what Dr. Matson said.

"Ear infection, my ass," Carol replied. "Mary Joe, I just talked to Mom. She is still nauseated and now she is vomiting. I told her not to take any more of those pills and I also called Dr. Matson to inform him of her symptoms. Mary Joe, I'm going to take Momma to another doctor the first of the week."

****

As I drifted back to the present, I felt Pat's arm tighten around my shoulder and I realized that, we four, Pat, Carol, James and I, were standing outside the hospital crying, huddled together each of us, I imagined wondering; 'Why? Oh, why did this cancer have nine months to grow? Oh. Oh. So sad. So sad.'

Pat wanted to know why Carol and I had left Mother's room.

"Pat, Mother was getting tired of us hovering over her since Tuesday. She wanted a little time to herself," I answered.

I let myself quietly contemplate, as the four of us walked back to her room, how Mother loved her family and, most times, was the one responsible for the family get-togethers. But she also liked her privacy and her independence. She would lose all this during the next four months, to her children and to those in the medical field.

Pat walked into Mother's room and quickly moved to the bed, falling into Mother's waiting arms. They were oblivious to all that was around them for that moment. Pat cried uncontrollably and Mother comforted her with her soft and loving words. Pat stayed the night; she told me later that she and Mother talked far into the wee hours of the morning.

I was up early Friday morning, as I wanted to get an estimate to remodel a room in my home. Thursday morning, the social worker at the hospital talked to Mother about alternatives available if she began to need constant care. She gave her several options at that time. They agreed that the two best options were: 1) She could return to her apartment and her children could take turns staying with her, 2) or she could move in with one of her children.

I had a two car garage that had been converted into a finished room. It had a bathroom and shower installed. Mother and I had talked about this as being a very workable solution. I knew that this would happen only if Mother was unable to remain at her apartment.

I called my good friend Paul, who was in construction, to come by and go over some changes to the room and give an estimate for what it would cost. We had worked together in construction for Raldon Homes as superintendents. If I had had the time, I could have done the work myself but there would be no time for me to even think about it. I knew I could depend on Paul if I had to get the room ready quickly.

I told Paul, "Mother loves the outdoors. I want to install a window that overlooks the back yard, put in a few cabinets and make a small kitchenette with a small bedroom off the large room. I want her to be able to have family members over to visit at her little apartment without having to come through my part of the house if they don't want to."

Paul let me know that he could do the work within a week if I needed to get it done. Mother wanted to remain independent and I wanted her to be able to for as long as she could. I knew that I would be only a door away from her and my plans were to install a direct intercom from her room to my bedroom in case she needed me at any time during the night. Then I would also be able to monitor her throughout the day as her illness progressed. But right now, I was working with a hypothetical situation. Mother's wishes, at this point, were to return to her apartment that she had lived in for the past ten years and to be close to her friends.

ANGEL IN DISGUISE

Three

Dr. Jones came into the room on Friday afternoon, October 6. Pat, Carol, James and I were with Mother and we knew that he would want to explain the treatments to all of us, as well as let Mother know when all the treatments should get under way. Dr. Jones explained about the radiation treatment that would be needed for the tumors in the head and about the chemotherapy treatments, which would be done in three phases.

Pat asked, "Why three chemotherapy treatments?"

Dr. Jones explained, "Chemotherapy is thought to kill a percentage of the total number of cancer cells. If the chemotherapeutic agents kill a percentage of the cancer cells each time, the third treatment your mother undergoes would make the cancer cell count considerably less. So, after several treatments, the number of cancer cells would be such that the immune system might, just might, be able to kill the last cells. But of course, the lung cancer is not the only cancer in your mother's body. The chemotherapy would have no major impact on the twelve tumorous brain cancers. In our bodies, there is what is known as a brain barrier and it is very selective as to what substances gets from the blood to the brain tissue. So, as I said, radiation is the best treatment for the brain tumors."

We asked other questions as he went through the methods and procedures concerning the treatments. When Dr. Jones finished, he asked if there were any other questions. There wasn't a word or sound from any of us. I wanted to get out of there and scream. 'Why? Oh, why is this happening?' I thought.

Mother sighed and began to speak. "I'll do the radiation treatments and I'll go through the three phases of chemotherapy but, Dr. Jones, if there is no improvement, I don't want to continue. I also want it understood here and now, there will be no, and I mean NO, intervention with machines to prolong my life if that becomes necessary, is that understood?" As she ended, with this question left hanging in the air, she looked from James, to Pat, to Carol and then to me, waiting for our response.

The four of us answered in unison, "If that's your wish, Mother. If that's your wish."

Dr. Jones acknowledged, "Mary Alice, it is your decision to make. I am here to help you, whatever you decide you want to do or not do."

Mother was released from the hospital on Saturday, October 7. She would begin the radiation treatment two days later.

On Monday, the radiation team at Methodist Hospital, led by Dr. Stevenson*, met with all of us including Carol's husband Dwight, who asked if he could be with us. He always felt that Mother was a second mother to him. They told us how many treatments would be needed and the procedure that would be followed for the thirteen doses of radiation that Mother would be given. This meant that, from Monday through Friday, Mother would need to be at the hospital's radiation department for her treatment. She would need one of us to be available to take her to these treatments.

Dr. Stevenson told us about the side affects that would probably be a result of the radiation. The main one was loss of appetite. He insisted that her meals consist of a balanced diet. In other words, the meals should be high in protein, high carbohydrate and low in fiber. We should take extra time to make the meals appealing, as Mother's sense of taste would lessen. Resting before and after meals would decrease her chances of being nauseated and/or vomiting. He said that she could experience some diarrhea and for that we would need to increase calories and fluids and provide a low roughage diet. The other side affect would be 'alopecia,' or, hair loss. He gave us the name of a shop that specialized in fitting cancer patients with a wig that is as close to the individual's hair as possible.

We were also precautioned against having Mother around a lot of people, as her immune system would become depressed and her white blood cell count might be low. He gave us the telephone number of the American Cancer Society should we need any support items to help with the care of Mother.

ANGEL IN DISGUISE

The radiotherapist came in and took us on a tour of the facilities. He described the steps that Mother would go through, from signing in for treatment, to seeing where she would be when they performed the radiation dosage. The radiotherapist told Mother that he would be stationed outside the treatment room where he would perform the treatment, and from there, he would be observing and in communication with her at all times. He explained that the treatment would last from one minute to two minutes. This would be determined by Dr. Stevenson after he reviewed Mother's medical records from Dr. Jones.

He then asked Mother to come into the room where she would be while the treatment was given. He asked her to clean her face thoroughly, then began to put marks (using a marker) on Mother's face and neck area. Mother was told that these marks would be his guide throughout the treatments. He advised her not to wash the marks off of her face during her baths until all treatments were finished. He told Mother that over the period of time he would be administering treatments, the rays would be directed at her from different angles to minimize the exposure to normal skin tissue. As I listened, my heart was burdened with what this wonderful woman was going to have to go through.

All I could think about was, 'I'll help you Mother. I'll do anything and everything that it takes to see you through all of this. I promise you. I promise you.'

Pat went along on a few of the treatments before

she had to go back to Texas City. I could see the fear and hurt that she was enduring as she said good-bye to Mother. "Please let me know if you need me to come back. I know I have my business to look after, but you are more important to me than any job or business. Please, Mother, promise me you'll do that," she said.

"I will, Pat," was her response.

It was up to Carol and me now to be with Mother on a continual basis at her apartment and to see that she had a way to the Cancer Radiation Department at Methodist Hospital.

By the time Mother had completed five of the thirteen treatments, there was a definite change in her eating habits. She had to be coaxed to eat. I knew it was important to keep her eating well-balanced meals, but there were times when she would say, "Mary Joe, I don't want to eat." She would push the food away with her hand, and when she did, I would pick up the fork and start to feed her. She would dart her eyes at me and say, "I told you I don't want this food."

"O.K. I'll fix you something else," I would reply.

"Don't get smart with me," was her answer.

"I know, Mother. You don't want anything to eat but you must, and I'm going to see that you do." That usually got her to go ahead and finish her meal. The struggle was always the same during each meal; to get her to eat enough to keep up her strength. My concern was that she still had eight more radiation treatments to go. The chemotherapy treatment would come and she would have to have her body built up for that procedure. I would think to myself, 'Mother, can't you see I'm not your enemy here.'

I made it a point to call Pat and keep her informed about Mother. During one of those calls, Pat told me about a night she had stayed with Mother. "I woke up and saw Mother walking out of her bedroom into the living room. She sat down in her rocking chair. I didn't say anything. Mother started crying. I started to say something to her but...I turned on my side, facing the other direction and thought, 'This is Mother's time for herself.' It was so hard to lay there and listen to her cry. She never knew I was awake."

On the sixth day of treatments, Mother and I left her apartment building and as we walked to my car, without any warning, Mother collapsed in my arms and I lowered her to the ground. Two of her friends saw what happened and rushed out to help me get Mother into the car. I still had a hospital parking lot permit designated for the cancer area parking, so, upon arriving at the hospital, I parked and went in to get a wheelchair for Mother. She was not able to make the walk to the department for her sixth treatment. After this incident, Mother never had the strength to walk on her own for any distance. She was able to use a walker for her trips to the bathroom which was located a few feet from her bed, but she needed the wheelchair on all other occasions. The American Cancer Society loaned us the support items we needed. Carol made the call to them and the response was prompt in getting the items to Mother that we needed for her care.

At first, Carol and I could leave Mother alone for a few hours, but now that she needed a wheelchair and walker, we no longer felt at ease leaving her even for a few minutes. So the time arrived when Mother would have one of her children with her at all times until the day she died.

Mother's last radiation treatment was on October 27. She put a twenty dollar bill into my hand and said, "Mary Joe, go over to the store and pick up two boxes of candy for the doctors and nurses. I want to show them that I appreciate what they've done for me."

"Just like her, thinking about what she can do for someone else," I kept repeating to myself as I made the walk to the store.

I also knew that I had an examination at school coming up in two weeks that I had not even started to review for. 'Maybe there will be time to study this weekend after Mother's last treatment,' I thought as I left the store and headed back to Mother's.

I had enrolled in the Nursing Degree Program at Texas Women's University a few months before we found out about Mother's illness. She was very happy that I had started to pursue my nursing education again. I had attended Arkansas Baptist School of Nursing back in 1955-1957, leaving school to get married. It was the policy of the school that you could not be married and stay in training. I knew Mother felt sad that I didn't finish at that time. I always felt she had wanted to be a nurse and, since she couldn't, she wanted me to be the 'nurse.' I had completed college, getting a Bachelor Degree in Business Administration, in 1975. I knew Mother was proud of that, but she had always hoped I would continue with my nursing education.

I didn't anticipate the demand that would be placed upon me and the rest of the family. To be a caregiver, you must be prepared to become more involved as the illness progresses. It was necessary for me to be in class, but as Mother's illness progressed, this became harder to do, so Carol and I juggled our time as primary caregivers. She had a contract to paint and wallpaper the living quarters of the priests of Saint Thomas* in Dallas. She was about halfway through when Mother's illness was first diagnosed. She would cover for me and I would do the same for her. Still, I realized that my schooling was suffering; I was missing some classes and when I tried to study at Mother's, I found it difficult.

I remember one particular Sunday: Mother was asleep and I was preparing for an examination. James had just left after spending Saturday night with Mother. I thought, 'Boy, I'll be able to get a lot of good studying in this afternoon.' WRONG!!

"Mary, could you come and help me to the bathroom?" She would call me in to take her to the bathroom, or to the living room, to sit and watch TV. This went on for the next four hours. Studying was out of the question.

The nights were getting worse as well. She would call me to help her to the bathroom. Just as I would start to drift off to sleep I would hear, "Mary Joe, Mary Joe, are you awake? Can you help me to the bathroom, again?" I know it was hard on her since she wasn't getting her hours of sleep, but neither was I.

"Mary Joe I need—."

"Oh, Mother, I love you so, but I need to get some sleep," I would say under my breath, but I would be up, in a flash, to meet her needs. I thought, 'I promised you I would take care of you during this battle. I won't break that promise to you, but this promise that I made, to myself, is not what keeps me going; it is the love I have for you and the wonderful example you have been for me, of how a person should live their life, to care about your neighbors and help those less fortunate. This is the way you lived your life, Mother; this is the way I remember you.'

****

One day I was approached by one of the residents at the apartment complex. Geraldine was a woman of color and was in a wheelchair. She began this way, "Mary Joe, you have the most wonderful mother that God put on this earth. Last month, I went out into the lobby to see if I could get help from one of the residents. I had lived in the high-rise for about two months and knew most everyone but really didn't know who I could depend on should I ever need any help. No one was there that I felt I could trust with my problem. I wheeled myself to the door of the crafts room and looked around and my eyes stopped on Mary Dee. I asked her if I could talk to her for a minute. She got up and came to the door. I began to tell her that it was two weeks before I would receive my Social Security check and I didn't have any food. I asked her if I could borrow some money until the first of the month. She said, 'Geraldine, meet me in my apartment in about thirty minutes. I need to clean up here before I leave.'

"When I got to her apartment, she opened the door and invited me in. Two sacks, full of groceries, sat on the table. She walked over and placed five dollars in my hand. 'Now you take the groceries. The money is to get something extra should you need it.'

"I told her, 'I will pay you back the groceries and the money when I get my check, Mary Dee.'

"She replied, 'You don't need to pay me back the groceries, Geraldine, but I would like the five dollars back.'

"As I left her apartment, loaded down with the sacks of food, she said, 'Geraldine, if you run short of food before pay day, you know where to come.'"

****

This was just one of many stories that I had heard over the years of living in the presence of this extraordinary woman. She was not a woman of financial means, but I do know that no one would ever go hungry if Mother knew that they were in need. Boy, could she cook and she always kept plenty of food in the pantry. I said many times, not really thinking of the reality, "If Mother ever dies, it must mean that God needs a good cook."

Four

Mother's body continued to weaken. I knew that this was not good for the upcoming chemotherapy treatment. Dr. Jones wanted to get under way as soon as possible after the radiation treatments were completed, so he scheduled chemotherapy to begin November 7. We had two weeks before that started. I found out that it was two weeks of an uphill battle with Mother to try to keep her eating the foods that would build up her body.

The treatment would take a toll on her body. The chemotherapeutic agents that destroy the cancer cells also destroy the good cells. That is the reason that she would probably start to lose her hair. Her leukocyte and thrombocyte count would also be at a drastically low point the seventh to fourteenth day after the chemotherapeutic agents were given. She would be at greater risk during this time for bleeding and infection, such as a respiratory infection. It would take about three weeks to get the count back up so that Mother would be ready for her second chemotherapy treatment.

Mother had been a smoker since she was twenty-five years old and was still smoking until she completed the radiation treatments, at which time, she stopped smoking. She might take a puff now and then, but after the chemotherapy she said she just didn't like the taste or smell. I remember that in 1987 I was over at her house and she began talking about wanting to stop smoking. I was surprised with this as I had always known her to be a smoker. She even stated that she might get in touch with my doctor, Dr. Waters, to see if he had some methods to help her stop smoking. To my knowledge, she never followed up on this, as she had continued to smoke up to this point.

Mother entered Northwest Hospital on November 7, to start the first phase of the chemotherapy treatments. She was upset that she could not walk into the hospital and fussed about being brought in by wheelchair. I could tell that she was very nervous. Alot had happened to Mother since she found out that she had cancer and this trip was one that would be started with needle sticks, obtaining blood samples, and proceed to the chemotherapy infusion being administered intravenously.

The only other time that I can remember Mother getting stuck with a needle was back in 1984, when she had developed an ear infection and I insisted on her seeing Dr. Waters. He did a routine office examination and told her that he was going to give her some medication that would clear up the infection. He left the room and Mother turned to me and said, "Mary Joe, where, where did he go?"

I told her he went to get the solution to give her a shot. When he came back, I told Mother that he was going to give her the shot in her buttocks. She reluctantly pulled her slacks down and then she held out her arms to me and I took her into my arms and stood there patting her on the back telling her everything was okay while Dr. Waters gave her the injection.

Immediately upon her admission to the hospital, Dr. Jones ordered an intravenous solution to be administered. He wanted to make sure that she was hydrated and that her kidneys were flushing urine for seven hours before starting the chemotherapeutic agents.

We were told that the chemotherapy treatments would be administered over a three day stay in the hospital. The antineoplastic agents that would be used in Mother's treatments were Etoposide (VP-16) and Cisplatin (Platinol). The first day would be VP-16, the second day VP-16 and Platinol, and day three, VP-16. Dr. Jones also ordered Phenergan, Reglan, and Decadron to be given for nausea and to reduce the pressure in her head due to the tumors. Mother began to complain of difficulty in breathing, so the doctor ordered respiratory treatments to be started on her.

Alupent was the medication of choice since the doctor wanted to dilate the bronchial tubes to get the sputum out of Mother's lungs. An arterial blood gas test was ordered and the findings showed that oxygen was low in her bloodstream, so oxygen was started right away at three liters/min. Mother didn't say anything while all this was going on. How could she; it seemed as though someone was working on her or getting her ready for a test ever since she was admitted. My heart was breaking seeing her this way. For a person who never had medical problems, this wonderful woman was having her share and then some.

I told Carol that I would remain with Mother the first night of her stay in the hospital. It was around six-thirty in the evening when the nurse came in to start the first chemotherapy agent (VP-16) intravenously. Mother got up and I helped her to the bathroom before the IV catheter was inserted. I noticed that she remained in there longer than usual. "Mother, are you all right?" I called out.

"Yes, I am Mary Joe, but let them wait until I'm ready and at this moment I'm not ready."

I knew that she was fearful about the treatments that she would be undertaking the next three days. How could she not be, with all that she had experienced during the radiation treatments.

When Mother started talking, it was more like yelling at me; "What's going to happen to me after these treatments? I don't want to eat, I'm losing my hair. Oh, Mary Joe, I'm so sick. Is this really worth it?"

I stood outside the door listening and found it hard to put together the words to answer her. 'Oh, Mother it's worth it!! If you weren't going through all this I couldn't talk to you on the phone, wouldn't see your face, couldn't kiss you or hug you.' All this raced through my head before I responded. "Yes, Mother, it's worth it." She opened the door and we stood there looking at each other.

Several hours later, after the IV had been started, Mother complained that her arm that the IV was in was hurting. No nurse had been in to check on Mother's progress since the chemotherapy treatment had been started. I felt that the nurse should come in and check on Mother. I knew from working with patients receiving chemotherapy that it's very important to closely monitor the IV, to check the IV flow and to check the skin around the catheter for redness, swelling, or drainage. In some cases, if certain chemotherapeutic agents are allowed to leak into the surrounding tissue, they could cause pain or destruction of skin, nerves or muscles. I felt it was about time that a nurse came and checked on MY MOTHER. I pushed the nurse call button.

The nurse came into the room and I explained Mother's arm was hurting and that I was concerned that no nurse had been in to check on the IV or how Mother might be tolerating the IV. The nurse appeared genuinely sorry for the way that I felt. We talked for a while, then she left the room.

It was late; Mother and I hadn't talk for quite a while. I looked over toward the bed and realized that she was asleep. I sat back into the chair and my eyes settled on the IV solution dripping and I thought, 'This is going into her veins. The solution will then become like a knight on a white horse out to slay the dragon (the cancerous cells) . . . What thoughts I do have these days.'

When the IV was just about finished, I rang the call button so a nurse would come in before the IV ran completely out. She and I talked while she waited for the remainder to run in. She then took out the IV catheter. 'Mother's first day of treatment is over,' I thought. I watched the nurse take down the bag that had contained the chemotherapy agents and throw it away in the trash can. She didn't wear special gloves for handling chemo products, nor did she secure the IV bag in a container marked specifically for disposal according to hospital policy. "Oh, god, who will be Mother's nurse for tomorrow's treatment and for those to follow?" I spoke under my breath.

The next day, I spoke to the supervisor about what had transpired and about my concern that there wasn't constant monitoring of the IV. I informed her, "I work in a hospital and know how busy the nurses can be. My sister and I bathe Mother and we change the linens on her bed. All we ask the staff to do is to furnish us with the items we need to care for her." The supervisor assured me she would handle the problem. I assumed she did, as the remaining two IV chemotherapy treatments given to Mother were continually observed and her vital signs periodically monitored.

After the first chemotherapy treatment, Mother urinated only 500 cc's of urine, so a Foley catheter was inserted into her bladder. Now she wouldn't have to exert herself to go to the bathroom. Also, from the time Mother was admitted to the hospital, medication was given routinely to keep her relaxed.

On the second day of admission she began to pick at the sheets and the air. "Mother, what are you doing?" I asked.

Her response was, "Nothing. Oh, nothing."

The day seemed to pass slowly and as night approached, I was ready to sit back in the recliner and relax. I knew Mother would be asleep before long and I would be able to get some sleep. The time came and I drifted off to sleep . . . but only for a few minutes. I woke up to the sound of rustling sheets. I jumped up from the chair and saw that Mother had scooted down to the foot of the bed. All the bed covers and her gown were off and she lay there 'stripped naked.'

"Mother, for heaven sake, what have you done?" I shouted.

"I'm not doing anything, am I?" she replied with a blank look in her eyes. Then I saw the catheter laying on the bed in a pool of blood.

"Oh, Mother, you've pulled the catheter out!"

"I did?" she said meekly.

I pushed the call bell to let the nurse know the catheter had been pulled out. The responding nurse said that she was going to wait until the doctor arrived in the morning to see if he wanted another one inserted. Why was Mother acting like this? I began to keep a closer watch on her movements.

Throughout the night and early morning, she seemed to be getting better. She was more in tune with her surroundings. Later, the nurse came in and inserted a continuous IV of medicated solution into Mother's veins. Within thirty minutes, Mother was picking at the sheets and the air again and she had that blank look in her eyes. I left the room and went to the nurses' desk to let the staff know of her change. Whatever medication was ordered to relax her might be having an adverse reaction. Dr. Jones discontinued the medication. For the rest of Mother's stay in the hospital, she was coherent.

Five

On Friday, November 10th, Mother was discharged from the hospital and instead of going back to her home, she went to Carol's house. Carol had decided it would be easier on all of us for Mother to be there. And from this time on, Mother never went back to her home of ten years.

Now it was up to Carol, James and I to take turns caring for her. Living three hundred miles away prevented Pat from helping us, but I knew, as did James and Carol, that Pat was always there; if not physically present, she was there in her heart.

Mother was back in control . . . or so Mother thought, since she had left the hospital. She was back to refusing to eat her food. She would let us know that she did not appreciate us trying to feed her. There were times that we even demanded that she eat, but, Mother would argue that she was not going to eat if she did not want to.

On Saturday, James went over to Carol's to take care of Mother. I went over on Sunday and stayed until Monday evening. I had made up my mind that I would bring my own meals to Carol's. I knew it was hard enough on Carol and her family to have Mother and one of us there all the time without having the responsibility of feeding us too. I had talked to Carol about this arrangement and she agreed to have coffee and tea available while I was there. She did mention that while James was there, she had to feed him.

I went home on Monday evening knowing that Mother wouldn't be able to come and live with me, so there was no need to remodel the garage into an apartment. I still wanted to be able to have Mother come over to my house and stay for short visits. It would give Carol a rest from the twenty-four hour activity going on at her house since Mother's arrival. I moved the furniture around in the front bedroom to accommodate Mother's wheelchair and walker. I was ready should Mother want to visit. How could I have known then that there would be no visit? The hospital and Carol's home would be the only places Mother would stay ever again.

On Tuesday, Carol let me know that Pat had called and was flying to Dallas to help with Mother. She was to arrive that evening, but a heavy fog moved into the Houston area and the plane wasn't able to leave until Wednesday morning. Carol picked her up at the airport. I knew Pat wanted to spend time with Mother, so I told Carol I would be over on Friday since I had to work at the hospital for the rest of the week.

I arrived about one o'clock. Carol had coffee and tea made. "Mary Joe, Pat and I are going to the Mall for the afternoon. I need to get out of the house for a while. Pat wants to buy a few sweatshirts. Momma didn't eat much for breakfast or lunch. Maybe you can get her to eat some oatmeal this afternoon. You know she loves oats."

"I'll do my best to get her to eat," I said.

I tried to feed her. She absolutely refused to eat.

Later, in the afternoon, she needed to use the toilet but the wheelchair was to wide too get into the bathroom. I lifted her out of the wheelchair and carried her to the toilet seat. It was almost impossible for one person to do because she couldn't use her legs to support herself at all. I had mentioned to Carol about getting a bedside commode; it would make it easier for us and for Mother.

Pat and Carol returned around five o'clock and I let them know Mother wouldn't eat no matter how hard I tried to encourage her. "It was a lost cause," I remarked. They left the room. Mother and I talked throughout the evening and many times during the night. At this point, clock time meant nothing. I slept when Mother slept and was awake when she was awake.

Saturday morning I noticed Mother had difficulty in carrying on a conversation. It was as though she was trying to figure out what to say before she would talk, or she would go blank in the middle of our conversation. I never pushed for an explanation about this. I guess I knew that twelve cancerous tumors in her brain would affect her communication skills. There were times when Mother would look straight into my eyes and make the comment, "So sad, so sad. Why, Mary Joe? Why?"

"I don't know, Mother. I just don't know." I assumed she was thinking, 'Why was the cancer not detected in December 1988.'

I left around noon on Saturday to go home. I had to work the next day. Pat said as I left, "Mary Joe, I'll call if there is a change in Mamma's condition."

As I drove home, I reflected back to Pat's statement; 'change in Mother's condition.' 'CANCER! That's her condition. What is going to change that? Will the treatments help? Oh, god, I hope so... but look at the toll the radiation treatments have had on her body.' I arrived home.

I needed to wash my uniforms and get them ready as I would be working a double shift on Sunday and the evening shift on Tuesday and Wednesday. Between caring for Mother and working and going to school, there was little time to do anything else. It was as though . . . my life was on hold.

That night before I went to bed I called Mother to tell her good night and that I loved her. Pat answered the phone.

"Pat, let me talk to Mother." She put the receiver to Mother's ear. "I wanted to talk to you before I went to sleep. I hope you sleep good tonight. Mother, I love you so much."

"I love you, too. Are you coming back over soon?" Mother replied.

"Yes, I'll be back over to see you real soon," I said.

A few days later, Pat told me that after Mother hung up the phone from my call, she turned to her and said, "Pat, I know you kids love me. Y'all have always told me that you loved me. This is not something y'all have just started saying to me because you know I'm sick."

On Monday morning, November 20, after getting out of class, I decided to stop at Carol's to see Mother before going on home. I knocked on the front door.

Dwight yelled out, "Door's unlocked, Mary Joe, come on in."

Pat was standing at the kitchen sink washing dishes and Dwight was in the den watching television.

"Hi, y'all," I said as I walked over to the table where Mother was sitting and gave her a kiss on the top of her head. She already had lost a lot of her beautiful gray hair and you could see her scalp. There was a dish of baby food in front of her. "When did Mother start eating baby food, Pat?" I asked as I walked into the kitchen area.

"Well, Mary Joe, she wasn't eating anything we fixed for her and I thought I would try her on some baby food. But she didn't eat that, either. I've been trying to get her to eat and, I hate to say this, but I forced her to eat a few bites." Pat stopped washing dishes and turned toward me. "Mary Joe, when I forced Mamma to eat she looked at me with tears in her eyes and said, 'Pat, my stomach hurts. I can't eat, please don't make me.' I felt so bad that I had forced her to eat those few bites."

I turned toward Mother. "If you don't start eating you're going to have to go back into the hospital."

Mother sat there in her wheelchair with her head down. She looked like a child being scolded. I walk-ed over and looked down at her; really looked... her skin color was gray and pallid. I took Mother's hand in mine and saw that the color under her finger nails was blue. She was cold and clammy to touch.

"Mother, how do you feel?"

"Mary Joe, I'm so sick. My stomach hurts real bad. I feel like I need to vomit."

I looked at Pat and Dwight. "Mother doesn't look good at all. I think we should do something."

Dwight spoke, "Do you think we should call the doctor or 911?"

"Let me call Dr. Thomas and let him know how she looks."

I called his office. "Dr. Thomas, I'm calling about my mother, Mary Davidson. This is Mary Joe. I'm over at my sister Carol's house. Mother is cold and clammy and her skin color is gray; she hasn't eaten very much since getting out of the hospital. She is complaining of her stomach hurting and she feels nauseated."

He told me to call 911 and to get her to the Emergency Room immediately. I hung up the phone and turned to Dwight, "Dr. Thomas said to call 911."

I dialed the number. For many years I have watched the television show, 'Rescue 911,' and now I was making that call. I gave the operator Mother's condition and our location. Within five minutes I heard the sirens and looked outside to see the ambulance and fire truck coming down the street. The Paramedics rushed into the house and lifted Mother out of the wheelchair and onto a stretcher. They began to take her blood pressure, pulse and respiration. They ran an electrocardiogram to check her heart while an oxygen mask was put over her face to give her pure oxygen. As they were wheeling her out to the ambulance, I asked where they were taking her.

"General Hospital," they told me.

"You can't take her to General," I said. I gave the paramedics a brief version of the problems Mother experienced there in December of 1988.

"Mother was in that hospital back in 1988 and because of what we view as a wrong diagnosis from the radiology department and her doctor, she is now in this condition."

Pat and Dwight both told them, "No way will we let you take her there."

They put Mother into the ambulance; I got into the front seat to make the trip with Mother. The driver made a call to 911 that he was taking Mother to Charter Hospital*, which was a little farther away.

I looked back into the ambulance where Mother was but I couldn't see her. I shouted out to her over the sounds of the siren, "Mother I'm here in the ambulance with you. We'll be at the hospital soon."

At eleven forty-five a.m. the ambulance backed into the Emergency Room driveway. From the time I called 911, to our arrival at the hospital, only twenty minutes had passed. I jumped out of the ambulance and ran toward the back. When I got there, the nurses were already taking Mother out of the ambulance. I looked at her face and could tell that she was terrified about what was taking place. I wasn't about to leave her side but I knew that the hospital staff would ask me to wait in the waiting room. When they did, I responded by saying, "I'm not going to leave my mother's side." The nurses didn't object, so I went into the emergency room with Mother, staying as close to the stretcher as I could in order to say out of the way of the medical team.

There were times when as many as six people were working on her at the same time. I was bent over, holding her hand and talking softly to her, trying to assure her that everything was going to be all right, and, more importantly, that I was there with her and wouldn't leave her alone! I didn't know if everything was going to be okay. So much had happened in the last two months since the diagnosis of cancer.

The emergency room doctor examined Mother immediately and asked me questions concerning Mother's health record. Then she ordered medications to be started. An intravenous solution was started to keep a vein open in case medication needed to be given through her vein. Mother was complaining of feeling pain above the abdominal area. Demerol was given for the pain. An electrocardiogram was taken to rule out any heart problems and the laboratory technician drew blood to do a complete blood work-up. A respiratory therapist drew blood for an arterial blood gas test. Oxygen was increased to three liters/min. once the blood gas results were known. A Foley catheter was inserted into her bladder for direct urine elimination. An x-ray was taken of her chest and the results showed she had pneumonia.

I wondered, 'What else is this woman going to have wrong with her?' The doctor inserted a Levine tube into Mother's stomach and suctioned out 500 cc's of old blood. To me it looked like coffee grounds. I now understood why she was in tears, complaining about her stomach pain. Exhausted from all the tests and procedures, the pain medication helped Mother to relax and she drifted off to sleep.

Pat and Dwight had followed the ambulance to the hospital and were in the waiting room when I walked in to let them know Mother's progress.

They wanted to go in and see her even though I informed them that she was asleep.

Pat went in anyway and when she returned, she was crying. "Mary Joe, I didn't realize Mamma was that sick. You know what I mean. All that blood in her stomach. And I forced her to eat. Oh, Mary Joe, I feel so bad about that."

"Pat, you couldn't have known that. Don't blame yourself."

"I'm so glad you came over this morning. What if I let Mother stay at the house that way? I didn't know. I just didn't know, Mary Joe."

As we stood there talking, Carol came rushing into the waiting room. "Mary Joe, Pat, how is Momma?"

"She's resting right now," Pat answered.

Carol went into the emergency room to see Mother and to let her know she was there. After several minutes, she returned. "You know, as I drove here, all I could think about was, 'am I going to be too late? Will Mother be dead when I get to the hospital?' I didn't think I could get here fast enough." We sat there discussing what had transpired throughout the morning.

At one o'clock Mother's condition had stabilized and the emergency room doctor called Dr. Thomas' office to inform him that Mother would be transferred to Northwest Medical Hospital to continue under his care. She was taken by ambulance and once again I rode with her. Pat and Carol followed in another vehicle. When we arrived at the hospital, Mother was taken directly to the Intensive Care Unit. This time, I was left standing at ... closed doors. This was one place the medical staff wouldn't let me stay by her side. She was now in their hands.

I turned to walk down the hall to the waiting room and there were Pat and Carol coming toward me. "They've taken Mother into the ICU and we'll have to wait until the nurses get her admitted. Then they'll let us in for a few minutes," I said.

At two-thirty we were able to go in to see Mother. James had arrived by that time, so the four of us walked into her room. There she was, lying on the bed with restraint straps around her wrists tying her to the bed. The nurse told us that Mother had pulled out the Levine tube that had been put in at Charter Hospital and she was trying to get out of bed. They felt that for Mother's own protection they needed to restrain her. I told the nurse that Mother had had adverse reactions to several medications during her last stay in the hospital. If the doctor had ordered Phenergan or Valium, they needed to let him know so he could discontinue them. I found out later that she was getting those medications and the doctor did discontinue them.

Once we left Mother's room I knew we must call her brothers and sisters to let them know what was happening. Pat and Carol left to make the calls.

When they came back, Pat said, "Aunt Joan will be here to be with Mother this Wednesday. Aunt Pauline will arrive on Thursday since that's the earliest flight she could get. I guess the airlines are busy with the Thanksgiving holiday this week."

We spent the rest of the day in the waiting room, taking turns visiting Mother at two hour intervals. Pat and Carol left the hospital at about ten o'clock. James and I, feeling completely exhausted, left at one o'clock a.m. to return later in the morning.

Pat and Carol arrived back at the hospital about seven a.m. It would be another hour before they could go in to see Mother so they decided to go down to the cafeteria and have coffee and a roll since they left home without eating breakfast.

At eight they returned and hurried into the ICU to Mother's room. The bed where Mother had lain the night before was empty and made-up. Pat grabbed Carol's arm, "My god, Carol, where is Mamma." They both rushed over to the nurses' desk.

"Where is my mother," yelled Carol.

"Who is your mother?" was the response from the nurse.

"Mary Davidson," both said in unison.

"Your mother was transferred to the second floor Medical Unit this morning."

Carol was angry. "That's pretty good. No one told us. We could have been with her." They went up to Mother's room. Pat called me to let me know Mother had been moved from the ICU to the Medical floor. I asked her if she had called James, since I knew he would be coming to the hospital that morning. She said she would call him.

Mother had not been responsive since her admission into the hospital. There were times that she could hear us and she knew we were there, but she wasn't communicating with us. Then there were times I knew she didn't know we were there.

Since Thursday was Thanksgiving, I told Pat and Carol I would spend Wednesday night with Mother. Her sister Joan had arrived from Arkansas and had also spent the night at the hospital. I could tell that she was very upset when she realized that Mother didn't know who she was or that she was there.

Thanksgiving Day was not what Pat had envisioned when she made her decision to spend this holiday with her family in Dallas. It had been seventeen years since Pat had been home during a holiday. When she married Jack, they spent holidays with his children from a previous marriage. Now, they were all grown and Pat thought it would be nice for all of us to be together during a holiday weekend. She informed us, back in June, that she and her family were going to be with us at Thanksgiving. This was three months before we knew Mother had cancer.

When I got over to Carol's house that afternoon, I could tell that this was not the usual joyous holiday we, as a family, had experienced over the years. While eating turkey and all the trimmings, my thoughts were of Mother lying there in the hospital bed and I started to cry. Mother was not here! She was terminally ill. I had to stop eating since I couldn't swallow the food; it seemed to lodge in my throat. Carol prepared plates of food for Mother and Joan. She knew that Mother wouldn't eat anything, but she wanted to take it there just in case.

Aunt Pauline arrived from Washington early in the afternoon and was anxious to go to the hospital to see Mother. After we all pitched in and cleaned the kitchen, Pat, Carol, Pauline and I went to the hospital. Mother was still unresponsive to our presence in the room. Over the next few days, we all took turns staying at the hospital with Mother.

Six

On November 27, the doctor told us that Mother would not survive another chemotherapy treatment. We now must remember Mother's wishes: "I'll do the treatments but, if there is no improvement, I don't want to continue and I don't want intervention with machines to prolong my life." We would now need to work with the doctor and the hospital social worker to engage a hospice agency to help us with Mother when she was ready to leave the hospital.

Mother became incontinent in regards to her bowel movements. I suggested to the nurse, rather than let Mother lie in her stool until she had a chance to attend to it, just supply us with the linens and we would clean her up. She made sure that we had plenty of diapers and linens.

When James arrived at the hospital to take care of Mother, I gave him an update on how she was doing. I was concerned about how he would deal with her incontinence. I told him, "If you hear Mother 'pass gas' she has probably had a bowel movement. Just call the nurse and she will clean Mother and change the linens."

The next morning, when Pat got to the hospital, James told her that he had cleaned and changed Mother himself. I knew from experience, working in a hospital, that women caregivers were the ones to perform such tasks. I have never been able to understand why most men won't accept the responsibility of total care for a loved one should a illness, such as this, occur within their family. I was so proud of James!

Later, that evening when the night nurse arrived, Pat asked, "My brother stayed with Mamma last night. How did he do?"

"He did just fine, I believe he slept through most of the night," she replied.

Pat told me later what the nurse had said. We both looked at each other. I shook my head, rolled my eyes and let out a sigh. We looked at each other again and broke into laughter, imagining James sound asleep as she made her nightly rounds. I never told anyone, not even James, about the night he stayed with Mother at the hospital.

Mother remained incontinent the rest of the week. With the additional care from her family she did not have a bed sore or breakdown of her skin. One of us was always right there to change her and keep her clean and dry. We also made sure we turned her from side to side and on to her back every two hours to prevent pressure sores.

On November 29, after the holiday, Pat returned to Texas City. James and Carol went back to work. I returned to school and also made arrangements with the hospital to work only on the weekends. It was back to juggling our lives, trying to maintain the normal everyday activities, while making sure one of us was always there to care for Mother. Aunt Pauline stayed in Dallas to help us in any way she could.

Carol met with the hospital social worker to hear her recommendation for a hospice agency in our area. She called Allcare*, a private hospice agency, to inquire about what she would need to do to get Mother into the Allcare Hospice Program. The administrator explained that a registered nurse would be assigned, who, working closely with her doctor, would meet all of Mother's medical needs while living in a home setting. A social worker would make home visits at least twice a week, to talk to mother and to counsel any other family members, if needed. A chaplain was on call at all times for spiritual support.

Three times a week, a nurse's aide would bathe Mother, help with her personal hygiene and change bed linens. Respiratory and physical therapists were available for treatments, if they were required. The cost of most medications and treatment would be paid for under the program. Since the hospice program is designed to allow a terminally ill person to die with dignity at home, the registered nurse would not call in a coroner or have an autopsy performed, as the law requires under other circumstances when a person dies at home.

The hospice program is not a final commitment. The family has the option of putting the patient back into the hospital if they find they need a rest. Also, the program can be discontinued if the family is too overwhelmed by the care involved for their loved one.

Pat returned to Dallas on December 9, but before she left on November 29, we, as a family, decided that it would be best to take care of Mother at Carol's home with the help from the hospice personnel. As Mother would be discharged soon, Carol arranged with the Allcare Hospice Agency to have a hospital bed, wheelchair, bedside commode and a respiratory therapy machine for her treatments of Proventil, to be delivered to her home before Mother's arrival. The day before her discharge, Carol asked for a Dobbler pump to assist in Mother's feeding since she was being fed through a tube in her nose going into her stomach.

Mother was responsive and knew that the decision she had made on October 6, not to continue treatment if there was no improvement, or if a complication arose, was now to be carried out by her children and loved ones. She never appeared to be afraid or fearful of the possibility that there was nothing else to be done except wait for death to happen.

In the middle of December she did make a request of Carol. "Please let me know daily as to what day it is and what is going on with the family and the world news. I don't want to lose touch with reality."

We made plans to go over to Mother's apartment to pack up her belongings and divide them among family members, according to Mother's wishes. Even though her apartment was small, she had the closet, shelves and corners jam-packed with things she had collected over the years. She was like a pack rat, always saving things, but she would often comment, "I've got to get rid of some of this stuff and get my apartment in order." Well, she never got around to doing that, and now, it was up to us to clear out the apartment and get rid of those very items she talked about. Some of her friends at the high-rise came to the apartment while we were there. It was hard to tell Mother's friends she would not be returning. They shed tears and so did we. It was wonderful to know she was so loved by so many.

Mother was discharged from the hospital on December 11. Pat rode in the ambulance with her to Carol's house. Carol went on ahead to check that everything was ready for Mother's arrival, and when she arrived, found the feeding pump wasn't there. She immediately called the Allcare Agency to find out where it was. They told her that the cost of the pump and Mother's insulin medication were not covered by the program because it was not considered essential for the direct treatment of her cancer. Carol told them everything that had happened to Mother was a result of her illness, be it the cancer or the medications she had to take because of the cancer.

Pat told me later that Carol was furious. She telephoned her U.S. Representative and Senator, who are responsible for government programs, and told them about Mother's illness and that she had just brought Mother home from the hospital to live out her last days there. Within the hour of Carol's call to her elected officials, Allcare called back and said that a feeding machine would be delivered and they also let her know all medications would be paid for.

Once we chose to put Mother into the hospice program, we immediately became her primary care-givers. It was up to us to take care of all her needs not met by the hospice people. But for a person to go into the hospice program the primary caregivers don't have to be family. A friend, volunteer or a medical person may be the caregiver. The person may also live in their own home or in a medical institution for the terminally ill.

Carol had converted two bedrooms into one large room a few years prior to all this. This room was a perfect place for Mother to be and for those who would be taking care of her. Carol had put a couch, coffee table and twin bed at the opposite end of the room from Mother's bed and television. The bathroom was located just across the hall. While Mother was awake we kept the television on for her. She had many programs she liked and we made sure those programs were on for her to watch. I believe, at least in the beginning, that she was aware of them and knew what was going on, but toward the end, I don't think so. We also played music that Mother liked. One night, Pat put the earphones on Mother and played a Kenny G. tape, 'Going Home.' Mother looked at Pat while it was playing and said, "Pretty. Louder! Pretty. Louder, louder!" Pat looked at Mother and began to cry.

Seven

Christmas was fourteen days away and Carol had already decorated the outside of her house with Christmas lights. Many times at night, when I was caring for Mother, I noticed her looking out the window at the lit-up lights. "Pretty, pretty," she would say.

Then, there were times during which she just stared out the window and said nothing. 'What is she thinking?' I wondered.

During the next few weeks she made the comment to each of us, "So sad. So sad. Why?"

"I don't know, Mother. I don't know, why," I would respond when I was with her. I didn't know why. I didn't have the answer to why the government had released radiation on thousands of us during World War II when we lived in Richland, Washington. I didn't have the answer to why Dr. Matson didn't put you back into the hospital in the early part of 1989 to find out why you weren't getting any better. I don't know why you have the cancer and why it wasn't detected sooner, but I do know this: it is sad . . . SO SAD.

Most of Mother's conversations had now become one liners.

"I don't know what you kids are going to do without me," she said to Pat one evening.

"We are grown adults, Mamma. We will be okay."

"I doubt it," was her reply.

No truer words were ever spoken. I still find myself wanting to seek out her counseling. I miss her so much and my life has changed dramatically based on how I now view my life in this world. I seek to know something about this planet I was born on. I take time to smell the flowers and to feel the earth under my feet as I walk my path of life. I don't plan on all those tomorrow's, but live each day hoping that when the day is over, I truly have lived it the best that I could, bringing happiness to myself and to others.

One evening Mother pulled the feeding tube out from her stomach. The nurse told us she wasn't going to restart it right away. She wanted to see if Mother would eat on her own. We now had to try and get her to eat. It took a lot of coaxing to get her to eat, but even at that, she never ate much. However, the feeding tube was never restarted.

It was about this time that Mother began to hallucinate. She would see things in the room. For instance, one day she told Pat, "Who does her hair?"

"What did you say?" Pat asked.

"Who does her hair?" repeated Mother.

Pat pointed to the television program that was on, thinking that Mother had seen someone on TV.

Mother told Pat, "No that person there."

"Here?" said Pat. She pointed to a balloon, on top of the television that had a picture of a wild bushy haired duck on it.

"Yes, who does her hair?"

Pat looked at Mother and couldn't help but break out into laughter.

It was several days before Christmas and I needed to shop for my two sons and three grand-children. I also wanted to buy a special gift for Mother. She was not going to be with us much longer; what would I choose for her that she could take with her. I remembered that, one day, several years ago when I was over at her apartment, she had asked me to go into her bedroom and get a particular box off the shelf. I brought it back into the living room. She asked me to open the box. "That pajama suit is what I want to be buried in," she told me.

I looked at her and said, "You had better write that request down and put it with your important papers. You will out live us all." At that time I really believed that.

'A bed jacket would be a perfect gift,' I thought. I headed to the Mall and after stopping in several lingerie departments, I discovered bed jackets were not a popular item. But I was determined to carry on with my quest and headed over to the Galleria. Macy's was not a store I shopped in very often, but, as luck had it, they had a selection of bed jackets. I spotted a beautiful pink quilted jacket, pulled the pajamas from their box and found they were a perfect match. A display of small satin pillows filled with potpourri were sitting next to the rack, and Natalie, who had gone shopping with me, bought one as a gift for Mother. As we were walking through the accessories department I saw a white silk turban. I thought, 'Pat might like to give this to Mother. It would cover what scant bit of hair she had left after her radiation and chemotherapy treatments.' So I added it to my purchases.

I began to cry right there in the store. I told Natalie, "These Christmas gifts, Mother will be taking with her."

Christmas day, a day of joy and celebration for most, was difficult for our family knowing that it would be our last Christmas with this precious individual.

We always took snapshots of the five of us when we all got together. Since my friend Natalie is a professional photographer, I had asked her if she would take a family portrait of us during the Thanksgiving Holiday. With Mother's radiation and chemotherapy treatments in progress, this plan had been canceled. I asked Natalie if she would take some pictures on Christmas Day, of us together with Mother. It would be difficult, knowing that it would be all that I would have left of Mother: memories on paper. But oh, how wonderful it is to look at them from time to time. A few weeks after Mother's funeral, I put together photo albums for Pat, Carol, and James, of the pictures that were taken. I still pull out my album to look at those pictures.

At Carol's, we opened gifts, took pictures and shared our Christmas meal. Mother drifted in and out of reality throughout the day.

When Erin and Shawn, her great-grandchildren, went into Mother's room to sing a couple of Christmas songs to her, a smile came over her face. We each took turns that day spending time with Mother, savoring the precious moments. It was with a heavy heart that I headed for home that evening.

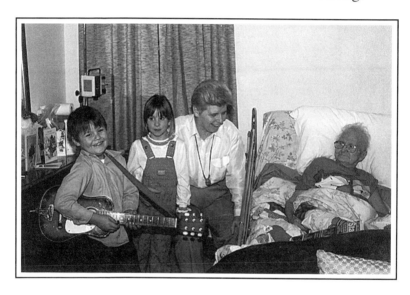

ANGEL IN DISGUISE

Eight

During the next week, there were times when Mother was coherent responsive to us, while at other times, her mind appeared to be somewhere else, carrying on conversations with those who we knew had died. One of these conversations stands out vividly in my mind.

She was talking to her brother Roy, who had died in 1974. She said, "Roy, Roy, don't leave me this time. Take me with you." She had been heard by others in the family talking to her mother and father. She even talked to my brother-in-law's mother, Beulah, and his sister, Beverly. They had died several years ago. Mother had known both of them.

A few days later, I was taking my dinner break at the hospital where I worked. I started to cry. One of the nurse's, who knew about Mother, asked me what was wrong.

I said, "I'm so envious of the ones waiting for her. She is closer to them now than she is to us."

Pat's family had come up for the Christmas holiday and needed to be home by December 30. We knew Pat wanted to spend as much time as she could with Mother before heading back to

Texas City. James and I also knew that, when Pat left, it would be up to us to help look after Mother. Time seemed to drag by in some ways, but in others it seem to fly by.

The day of Pat's departure arrived. It was hard for her, as she felt it would be the last time she would see her Mother alive. She went into the room to tell Mother good-bye. Sitting down on the edge of the bed, she said, "Mamma, hold me." Mother reached out and put her arms around Pat. They sat there, holding tightly to each other. "Mamma, I have to go back to Texas City, but I want to tell you that you have been a wonderful mamma and I love you so much. I have loved you more than I could ever tell you in words."

Mother replied, "You have been a wonderful daughter, too, Pat, and I love you."

At those words, Pat broke down and sobbed openly. Mother held Pat to her breast. During the past few weeks there were times when Mother was disoriented or confused and didn't recognize those around her. Pat was so happy when Mother called out her name. Mother knew who she was: 'PAT.'

After Pat left, James and I took turns going over to care for Mother. I would stay at Carol's for twenty-four to thirty-six hour interval's to give Carol and Aunt Pauline a rest.

I knew it was hard for Carol to take time for herself even when James or I was there, but it was important for her to be able to spend time with her own family, to relax, or be able to leave the house and run errands. As I said earlier, Carol had made the room comfortable for another person to stay and sleep in. I can't express in words how much I appreciated my sister and her family for allowing our mother to live and die with dignity in their home. Carol had installed an intercom system in the room so she could hear Mother anywhere in the house. We could even monitor her breathing.

We continued to take turns with Mother for the next ten days until it was time for Aunt Pauline to go back to Washington. She needed to return home, having been with us since November 23rd. She said her final good-bye's to Mother knowing that it would be the last time she would see her sister alive. She told us it would be too expensive for her to come back for the funeral.

On Saturday, January 13, Carol called to let me know Mother had stopped eating on Friday morning and she hadn't eaten since and wouldn't even drink water. I asked if I should come over, but she said, "Since you're coming over on Sunday to take care of Momma, I don't think that would be necessary. If I can't get her to eat, I don't think you could."

Later that day, I called from work to see how things were with Mother. "Carol, how is Mother doing," I asked.

"Oh, Mary Joe, while the nurse was here earlier, Mother began coughing. The nurse handed her a Kleenex and Momma coughed up a clot of blood. She looked down and when she saw the blood, there was such a sad look in her eyes. After the nurse left, Momma turned to me and said, 'Why? Why did this have to happen to me?' I shook my head and asked her if she wanted me to read the Lord's Prayer. She nodded yes. I read it to her word for word. Sometimes I just don't know how to answer Momma."

"I know what you mean," I responded.

On Sunday morning I called Carol to tell her that I'd be over at four o'clock. "Mother's friends, Liz and Marie, are coming over at six. Why don't you wait and come over after their visit," replied Carol.

"Okay, that sounds good. It'll give them some time to be alone with Mother." At seven-thirty that evening I called back. "Carol are they still there?"

"Yes, Mary Joe, but come on over anyway. I'm going to the airport later to pick up Pat. She's arriving at ten o'clock."

I was puzzled. 'Pat's coming back? Why? What was going on?' I thought to myself as I got ready to leave my house. I had been at work for the last four days and hadn't seen Mother at all during that time.

When I arrived at eight, Carol said, "Momma still hasn't eaten or had any water. She's getting worse. I called Pat this afternoon after I talked to you, to let her know about Momma. She called me back within a half hour to let me know she already had purchased a plane ticket and would be arriving in Dallas at ten o'clock. I've called James and told him about Momma's deteriorating condition. I knew you were coming over, so I decided to fill you in on all that was happening when you got here."

We talked for a while until Liz and Carol left for the airport to get Pat.

I tried to get Mother to drink some water, but she would just turn her head away when I put the glass up to her lips. I told her, "Mother, you must start eating and drinking some liquids." There was no response from her.

At eleven o'clock, Pat arrived. We all talked about the fact that Mother must start eating, but we knew in our hearts that Mother's time with us was coming to an end. She had lost so much weight that, I'm sure, at that time, she couldn't have weighed more than 90 lbs.

We talked for a while longer. Liz and Marie said their good-byes, saying they would be back on Wednesday evening.

ANGEL IN DISGUISE

Nine

At one-thirty a.m. on Monday, January 15, James arrived. All of Mother's children were with her now. We began a vigil without realizing it at the time. James and I sat on opposite sides of Mother's bed. Pat and Carol sat on the couch and talked for a while. Then they bedded down for the night, on the couch and bed located at the opposite end of the room.

James and I talked throughout the night and when Mother would wake up we always let her know, "We're all here with you, Mother. Your kids are with you. Mother, we love you, but you already know that." She was so weak but she would manage or try to say, "I love y'all too."

Monday morning Carol and Pat woke up around eight o'clock and went into the kitchen to fix breakfast. Pat brought James and me a plate of food, while Carol made a telephone call to the registered nurse to give her an update on Mother's condition. The nurse told Carol she would be over to the house later that morning.

Pat and Carol took this time to take their bath and straighten up Mother's room. I gave Mother a sponge bath and changed her bed linens. I asked her if she would eat some oatmeal and she nodded her head, yes. I no sooner got the words out of my mouth when the nurse arrived.

The nurse listened to Mother's heart through the stethoscope and informed us the beat was quite rapid, one hundred and fifty beats a minute. She told us it would only be a matter of time before Mother died and not to force her to eat or drink. She pulled out a bottle of Roxanall (morphine) and explained how to place the drops under Mother's tongue with a medicine dropper. "Give 1/2 cc at a time. Don't worry about giving her any of her other medications. Increase the dose if the 1/2 cc doesn't keep her relaxed and comfortable. The purpose of this medication is to let her go with as little pain as possible."

"What if I give her too much," Pat asked. I could tell Pat was still uncomfortable about giving Mother medicine.

"Then she will simply go to sleep and not wake up. She will just die," was the nurse's answer. "Do you all want me to stay for a while."

Carol answered, "No, I believe we'll be okay for now. We might need you later on. I know you told me you would be available day or night should I need your help."

Later Monday morning, James called work and I heard him say, "My mother is dying. I'll be with her until she is gone. If you need to talk to me, this is the phone number where you can reach me." I had already laid down on the bed to try and get some sleep when he came back into the room. I told him that evening would come sooner than we realized and we needed to be ready to care for Mother throughout the night. He lay down on the couch and soon we were both asleep.

Pat woke us at seven o'clock that evening. I got up and went into the bathroom to take a shower and freshen up before James and I took over Mother's care. Pat brought some food into the bedroom and we ate, but each bite was hard for me to swallow. My thoughts went back to the morning. 'Oh, Mother, you wanted some oatmeal but the nurse arrived and I forgot about it. But, would you have eaten it? Mother, Mother, I'm so sorry I forgot.' I began to sob aloud. James looked over at me but didn't say anything. I guess he was in his own world of thoughts.

I called the hospital where I worked and told them, "I will be with my mother until she dies. She hasn't eaten or had anything to drink for four days. I don't think it will be much longer before she is gone but until that happens, I want to be with her for as long as I can."

I hung up the phone, turned and looked at Mother and then at Carol, Pat, and James. There we were, the five of us, one waiting for death and the four of us watching, loving, touching, talking to this woman whom we had loved and known for the entirety of our lives as MOTHER.

Carol's family took on the responsibility of feeding us. They were wonderful and I knew it was a strain on them. They, too, loved Mother dearly.

We were each in our own world of memories as well as constantly thinking ahead of what we might say to Mother when she awoke. Now that we were giving her the morphine under her tongue, there were three to four hour periods of time that she would be asleep. The only thing we requested from each other was, "If I'm asleep when Mother wakes up, wake me up! I want to be able to talk to her and see her." Sometimes it seemed she recognized us and then sometimes I knew she didn't.

During Monday night and the early Tuesday morning hours, James and I sat up to care for Mother. Each time she awoke we would wake Pat and Carol. We all stood around the bed talking, crying, touching and holding her. Then, when it looked as if Mother was getting anxious or agitated, we would look at each other, crying, and say, "We need to give her the morphine." It was so hard to do because she would then go back to sleep. We were very selfish of her time now, but it was all we had left. I wanted to keep her awake for as long as I could, just to be able to look into her eyes and have her see me. When the morphine took affect, her eyes would close.

My niece, Ginger, had given Mother a little cross the last time she was in the hospital. James had placed it on Mother's chest. It wasn't on a chain so each of us had to continually place it on her chest when it slipped off. Carol had brought her a little white Bible during this time and Mother held it constantly, except for the times Carol would take it and read scripture to her.

Mother had never talked to me about her religious beliefs, although I knew she was a member of the Methodist Church. She wasn't a church goer, but the way she lived her life was one filled with caring and compassion for others. As little as Mother had, there was always something she had to give to those who had less than herself.

Eight o'clock, Tuesday morning, Pat and Carol were up and getting ready to start the day caring for Mother while James and I thought of getting some sleep. We both knew that sleep for us was only while this loving person had her eyes closed. When her eyes opened, Pat or Carol would wake us so we could be right there by her bedside, getting one more treasured moment with Mother.

During the day the nurse came to see Mother. After listening to her heart and getting updated from Pat and Carol, the nurse commented, "It won't be long, but I've said that before and look at how long she has lasted. It is impossible to give a certain time for death. When it's time, it happens." She stayed for a while talking with Pat and Carol, letting them know, once again, that she was available day or night.

James and I lay down and were soon asleep, but throughout the rest of the day we were awakened twice by Pat or Carol. Every once in a while Pat or Carol would leave the room to take a smoke break. They felt it best not to smoke in Mother's room because of her condition but, also, because James and I were non-smokers. Sleep came in fits for all of us. We all knew time was running out and we reached for and held onto those precious moments we had left to be able to talk and be with Mother.

Before she tried to go to sleep that night, Pat told me that on several occasions, she noticed Mother had put her finger between the pages of the little white Bible and even though Mother appeared to be asleep, Pat said she could hear Mother say, "Uh, huh." She told me, "It was like Mamma was hearing someone speak and it had to do with what was on those pages in the Bible. She did this several times throughout the day."

Wednesday morning Mother's brothers and sister called from Arkansas to see what was going on. We told them they might want to stay close to their home since we would probably be calling them soon to let them know that Mother had passed on. They expected as much but each of them were still in disbelief that their sister was this ill. Their mother, Annie, had lived to be ninety-one. I guess they thought Mother would do the same. I know I had thought she might outlive some of us, her own children.

Later in the evening, Liz and Marie came over to see Mother and to be with us. Before they left we said a prayer led by Liz. I remember as if it were yesterday she said, "Lord comfort Mary's family. Show them, Lord, your mighty powers."

Ten

On Thursday morning, January 18 at about three o'clock, Mother woke up. James woke up Pat and Carol and said, "Mom is awake and it looks like she might know what is going on."

Both of them jumped up and ran over to Mother's bed. They talked to her, "Mamma, we love you."

In a low, muffled voice, she said "I wove wo, too."

We all knew what she said even though the pronunciation was incorrect. She tried turning her head in an effort to look at each one of us but it was a strain for her to do this. James said, "Let's stand at the foot of the bed so Mother doesn't have to turn her head." So, there we stood, all of us looking at our Mother, and she, looking at us . . . AT ME. We were all talking and crying at the same time.

"Mother, tell us good-bye," we said in unison but she didn't respond.

Then James spoke, "Momma, if you're not going to tell us good-bye, give us that sweet little smile we all know."

My mother SMILED . . . We broke down again, crying openly. What a smile! I will never forget it. My heart was joyful and breaking at the same time.

We talked to Mother for a while longer, then her left arm began to jerk quite rapidly. We looked at each other, knowing it was time to give Mother the morphine. We were crying uncontrollably knowing we had to give it, but wanting this moment of being close again with Mother to last. Pat, with tears streaming down her face, gave the morphine drops, while Carol ran into the bathroom and brought four washcloths, one for each of us. There we four stood, at the foot of the bed, crying and telling Mother we loved her. Mother lay there in her bed looking at us . . . and then . . . her eyes closed.

That was the last time Mother was responsive to us. Even though Mother's eyes were closed, we always talked to her, hoping beyond all hope, that she might hear us and know that we were there.

Pat and Carol didn't go back to bed. Mother's condition began to change drastically over the next few hours. Her breathing became shallow and uneven, more like gulping for air. I picked up the stethoscope and listened to Mother's heart beat. The count was down to about forty beats a minute. I told the others. They leaned over the bed, hovering over Mother, realizing that the end was near. I kept the stethoscope ear piece in my ears. MOTHER'S HEART STOPPED beating. I yelled at the others, "Her heart has stopped!!"

I jerked the stethoscope off and grabbed for any part of Mother that I could latch on to, screaming, "Mamma, Mamma, Mammaaa." I couldn't see anything as my eyes were so full of tears.

Even over my own screams, I could hear James, Pat and Carol crying and screaming Mother's name, as well as feel Mother's body being tugged by them. We had said we were ready to let her go, but when Mother's heart stopped beating, we grabbed for her body. There we were crying and desperately holding on to her.

Several minutes went by and there seemed to be no end to the crying and grabbing by each of us, for Mother's body. All of the sudden, I heard a heavy sigh . . . COMING from Mother? I looked down. Mother was BACK . . . BREATHING again. I could not believe it!! SHE WAS BACK!! And we said we were ready to let her go. I think not.

Later that morning we talked about what had happened just a few hours earlier. We knew that eventually we were going to have to let Mother go, but we couldn't bring ourselves to say, "Yes, we're ready to let her go." Carol took hold of Mother's left hand and I took hold of her right hand. Then we joined hands with James and Pat and created a family circle; a circle that would be broken only by the death of our MOTHER. Each one of us stood there and one by one, made the commitment to let Mother go.

I lay down on the bed and was able to sleep for a few hours. When I awoke, I walked over and sat down in the chair next to her. I just wanted to be near Mother.

ANGEL IN DISGUISE

Eleven

I was standing near the window watching the rain come down. It had been raining for the past two days. I looked over at Mother, then back outside. "They are crying in Heaven for Mother," I said out loud. I looked at Pat. She glanced up with a puzzled look on her face. "The rain is really tears," I said as I turned, once again, to look outside. I didn't say anything else and Pat didn't comment on what I had said. But, what else needed to be said?

It was about three o'clock in the afternoon and the rain had stopped. I was sitting on the couch and Pat was sitting next to Mother. Carol's dog, Saber, came into the room and went over to the left side of the bed. She laid her head on the edge and looked at Mother. Pat said, "What's the matter, Saber?" I looked over at Saber and saw she was shivering. Pat called her over and gave her some pats. The dog looked over at Mother and walked out of the room. "I wonder what was wrong with Saber," Pat repeated.

Natalie arrived about four-thirty in the after-noon. She tried to get over or call at least every other day to see if we needed anything or to run any errands for us. I talked to her about what had happened to Mother that morning.

Natalie told me about something strange that had happened Monday evening: "Sabrina, a woman that I had met through a spiritual workshop, called me. We'd both moved since seeing each other last and had lost contact with each other during the past year. Sabrina, now living in California, had gotten my phone number from a mutual friend in New York. For some reason, during our conversation, I told her, 'Mary Joe's mother is dying and she has been with her, at her sister's, since Sunday.'

"Sabrina told me she has been with several people when the spirit has passed on. She explained that it's quite a remarkable experience to be there but it's important to let the spirit go, as it no longer needs the physical body. If the spirit is not able to leave when the time comes, it becomes painful for that physical body.

"Then, I told her, I would pass that on to Mary Joe and said it was good hearing from her."

I then told Natalie how James, Pat, Carol and I joined hands with each other and with Mother and made the commitment to let Mother go the next time she tried to pass on.

"Natalie, she was gone, free from all pain forever. We might have been responsible for bringing her back through our grabbing and holding on to her physical body and not letting her spirit pass on."

We talked for a while longer, then I left the living room and went back into Mother's room.

Twelve

NOTE TO THE READER: These moments are impossible to speak of as if they are in the past; they still feel really 'present' nearly four years later, so I have written of these events in the present.

I have used italics to set apart the extraordinary events that I, and my family, witnessed during those five-and-one-half hours, from my narration of the ordinary events. Where Pat or Carol are telling what they saw from their own point of view, I have begun the paragraph with the speakers name in parenthesis. In these italicized sections, the pronoun 'I' refers to the person who is recounting her experience.

As I write what happened over the next five and one half hours in Mother's room I feel as if I'm there again.

ANGEL IN DISGUISE

(Mary Joe)

Pat and James are sitting on either side of Mother's bed. Carol is sitting on the ottoman, and I'm standing at the foot of the bed to the left of Carol. The room is dark except for a small light on the dresser behind James. It is about five o'clock and already getting dark outside. Mother is gulping for every bit of air she can get into her lungs. It is so hard watching and I am full of conflicting emotions while witnessing her battle to hang on to life.

My eyes are filled with the full image of my mother lying there on the bed. Her body is stiff and rigid; her head is arched back and pressed deep into the pillow. It is so quiet.

I begin to see movement above Mother's body. 'What in the world is going on?' I think. Then all of a sudden Mother's bed is all lit up with rays of gold and crystal clear light radiating on, above and around the bed. My mouth opens in amazement at what is happening. I can't believe what I'm seeing . . . but I don't know what I'm seeing I see all this going on and I see Mother's body lying there. Then this electrical like activity becomes so intense that I can't see Mother's body anymore.

I leave the room and rush down the hallway to the living room where Natalie is sitting on the couch. "Natalie, something's happening in Mother's room. I'm seeing rays of light everywhere and one time I couldn't see Mother because of light streaking all above her body. What do you think it is?"

"I don't know. But whatever it is, go back in there and be open to what you're seeing."

(Mary Joe)

I hurry back into the room and stand at the foot of the bed hoping and wondering, if what I saw, just moments before, was going to happen again. I don't have to wait long for the answer.

The wall behind Mother is no longer a wall. There are no corners or ceiling in view. It's as though I'm standing back and looking into an area that has infinite depth. Behind, above and on both sides of Mother glows the whitest white light I have ever seen. I look at Mother and see, illuminating the top of her head, an aura-like halo. Then as I look straight ahead into the white light, bands of gold appear in the distance. From where I'm standing, in front of me, the area is lit up with this brilliant array of white light and gold, bright but relaxing to my eyes. I'm in awe of what is happening. I know that what I'm seeing is not of this world but I'm not afraid.

My eyes settle back on Mother. In a flash, there are beams of crystal clear light shooting outward in all directions from an area centered above Mother. In between the beams there are numerous round objects, like the tops of people's heads. With all this energy going on I can't see Mother on the bed and feel my heartbeat racing out of control; it is pounding fast and loud. There is Mother's body again. I can see her. Oh, what is going on? It's as though I'm in a trance. There is movement going on just above Mother. I look really hard to see what it is but I don't have to. It shows me. My mother's spirit moves to the left of her body and floats over to the edge of the bed. It then shoots back above her body.

I gasp, turn and run out of the room and down the hallway to where Natalie is. "Natalie, I'm seeing white light everywhere and I just saw Mother's spirit. I could see Mother's body and could see her to the left of herself. You know I'm not crazy, but what I'm seeing no one, I mean *no one*, is supposed to be able to see!"

"Who said?" she replied.

I paused and said, "I don't know." With that response, I ran down the hallway and back into the room.

(Mary Joe)

Am I going to have the privilege of seeing anymore of the magnificent scenes I have already been blessed to witness? The answer is YES. Moments after getting back into the room, the spectacular events begin to unfold again. Movement over Mother; I get to see more!! The force responsible for what is going on in that room is like a magnet drawing me more and more into the splendor of each glorious moment that my eyes behold. Mother's spirit is on the move. It glides over the bed with such ease, going to the right of her body and to left, always stopping at the edge. Several more times, Mother's body is blocked from my view by the voltaic energy exploding, shooting beams of crystal clear light and gold streaks across and above her bed. Activity is accelerating as I move into this majestic drama being played out in front of me. The star is Mary Alice Davidson. The director is her Lord. I am a spectator for this one time showing and I have a front row seat.

So far, I haven't said anything to the others in the room. 'Should I say something to them about what I'm seeing? What if I don't and Mother dies and then I tell them? Will they be mad or upset?' All this is racing through my mind as I watch the spirit move freely over the bed.

(Pat)
I notice Mary Joe leave the room a couple of times and then return. I watch her, her mouth and eyes open wide like she is surprised or as if she sees something. I think 'What is she doing?'

Finally I have to speak up. "I don't know whether I should say this or not because y'all are going to think I'm crazy, but I have to tell y'all what I'm seeing. I'm seeing Mother's SPIRIT. It's about six inches above Mother. I've watched it go from the left to the right side of Mother to the edge of the bed. Sometimes in a flash it returns hovering directly over Mother."

"That's nice, Mary Joe, but all I see is my mother's body," James said.

James, Pat and Carol leave the room.

I know they have left the room but it is as if they are apart from me and where I am. I am drawn to the action taking place in front of me. I don't want to lose sight of my Mother's spirit or lose the restful feeling that is within me. It is like standing on the edge of the world looking into another dimension.

(Pat)

The three of us leave Mother's room and go into the kitchen. James begins to tell Jack, "Mary Joe's in there saying she sees Mother's spirit."

Pat said, "Well James, you never can tell. Maybe she does."

"I'm not saying that she doesn't see something, Pat. I guess people can see what they want to see. But all I see is Mother lying there."

"Well, I haven't seen anything and I want to get back in there," I say, as I head down the hall.

(Mary Joe)

I'm not aware of when they come back. I know I was watching the spirit drifting over to the left edge of the bed. Up until now all activity has been confined on, above or around the bed.

I said, "Pat, she's coming toward you."

This time the spirit doesn't stop at the edge. In a split second, the SPIRIT soars off the bed. I'm startled by what I see. It leaves the bed in the form of a perfect square. The background, inside the square, is the whitest white I have ever seen and within this square is a face with dark eyes and long, wavy hair. The SPIRIT is looking straight at me with piercing but tender eyes. The mouth is shaped like a triangle. The spirit darts behind Pat who is sitting in a chair beside the bed. "Pat, the SPIRIT is behind you," I shout.

(Pat)

I jerk my head around toward the back, but all I see is the wall. I think to myself, 'What in the world is Mary Joe talking about?'

(Mary Joe)
Unbelievable things are happening before my eyes. The spirit goes behind Pat but now it's there in front of her chest. The face inside the square is looking at me. The mouth is moving as though it's talking to me. The spirit looks happy. A feeling of contentment flows through my body. 'This beautiful face is having fun with me,' I think.

"Pat, the SPIRIT is in your chest." She looks down at her chest, and sees . . . Nothing!!

I'm looking at Pat. There is a brightness about her. I stare in wonder at what I see. Pat's body is completely enclosed with the white light. I can see the light at Pat's feet. But how is that possible? The bed is in the way. My eyes can see everything on this stage that is lit up. Even when I look directly at Mother, I can see James and Pat sitting to the right and to the left of Mother as if I'm looking straight at them. What wondrous scenes I am able to gaze upon.

'All this is impossible and must be heaven at work,' is the thought racing through my mind and yet my mind is free from all but what I'm experiencing.

This pageant isn't for my eyes only. The other spectators have arrived and take their seats to behold this grand drama.

(Pat)
I look at Mother. There is a haze directly over Mother's body. I look around to see if anyone has been smoking in the room. No, it isn't cigarette smoke. I look toward an open window to see if

dust is coming in. No, it isn't dust. Then I look back at Mother and see rolling clouds of mist pouring from her nostrils and mouth. I watch the mist travel down toward Mother's feet and settle above the length of her body.

"Carol, get over in my chair and look above Mamma," I scream as I jump from the chair and head for the hallway, grabbing Mary Joe by the collar as I ran by.

"What you're seeing, is it like a haze over Mamma? Like cigarette smoke?"

"No, Pat. I see Mother's spirit lying above but next to her."

"I don't see that."

When we return to the room Carol is jumping out of the chair, yelling, "James, get over here and look above Momma."

(Carol)

I see a haze over Mother. James hurries over and looks above Mother's body. "I don't see anything," he responds, returning to the chair where he had been sitting.

I am ecstatic. Pat and Carol had seen something!! I sit down in the chair to the left of Mother to see if I can perceive what it is Pat and Carol have witnessed. I don't. Pat stands at the foot of the bed with Carol sitting on the ottoman to the right of Pat.

(Pat)

*I look at Mother. Nothing! I look again. Nothing!
I think to myself, 'Well, whatever Mary Joe is seeing
I'm not.' I look again hopefully for a third time.*

*At about this time, directly in front of me, the
room lights up with white and gold light, and there
is movement above Mamma. I'm hypnotized to what
is going on. I move closer to the foot of Mamma's
bed and notice that the room is getting larger and
wider and that the light is brighter. Mamma is lying
on the bed. Beams of light are shooting all over the
top of the bed.*

Pat begins to cry, tears running down her face.
With her arms outstretched and hands clutched tightly
she says, "Oh, sweet Jesus, sweet Jesus." I know she
is seeing something majestic. The moment is broken
for me by the movement of James leaving the room.
Evidently, this is not the case for Pat; it seems she
is in a world of her own.

Carol moves over into James's chair. I am sitting
to the left of Mother. Pat is not saying anything to
us but I can tell from her facial expressions that
she is still seeing something.

(Pat)

*I'm watching the activity happening in front of me
but I can see Carol all lit up with an aura from the
top of her head to her feet forming a complete outline
of her body. Carol is wearing a red outfit and Mary
Joe has on black Mary Joe is engulfed in a bright
light from head to toe. I look closer at Mamma; gray-
ish light and streaks of silver are shooting in all direc-*

tions above and around the edge of the bed. Mamma has a bright light around her head.

I have to get back to the foot of the bed where the best seats in the theater are, so to speak. James has come back into the room and he and Carol are standing together at the left side of Mother with Pat remaining at the foot of the bed along with me.

(Mary Joe)
"Carol, Mother's spirit is moving toward you," I say. Carol has her right hand resting on Mother's arm. "Carol, the SPIRIT is traveling up your arm. Oh, Carol you are cradling the spirit in your arm." What an incredible sight; Carol holding onto Mother's arm and cradling the spirit at the same time.

(Carol)
I look down and see a bright light near my elbow. I see the upper part of a face with dark, hollow eyes and nose. The hair appears to be flaming, white light.

(Mary Joe)
"James, the spirit is coming towards you. It's off the bed going up your arm." The spirit shoots off the bed in a flash, and is once more in the form of a perfect square. Inside the square is a brilliant white background. And the face, the face is there!! Oh, God, I get to see that precious face once more. Those beautiful dark, piercing eyes are looking at me. Oh, how wonderful it makes me feel. I feel so close and connected to this divine spiritual being. My eyes are focused on nothing else but the face,

dark nose, the dark triangular shaped mouth and the long, wavy, dark hair.

The spirit travels up James arm and then, almost as if it knew it had come to his heart, it stops. "James, the SPIRIT is in your heart," I whisper, as tears fall from my chin. Its little mouth is moving as if talking to me and deep within myself, I know it is saying, 'Oh, Mary Joe, this is so peaceful. I feel so alive and free.'

I believe I could live the rest of my life in this splendor. I want it to keep going on and on.

(Carol)

All is quiet in the room. My eyes are on my wonderful and loving mother. I glance outside; it is dark and sprinkling rain. It won't be long before Aunt Pauline's plane arrives. She had just left less than two weeks ago and said she wouldn't be able to come back for the funeral, but when I called her on Monday to let her know Momma's condition, she told me she was coming back. Richard is probably already at the airport to pick her up.

I turn back to Momma. 'Hang on, Momma, just hand on. Aunt Pauline will be here soon.' These thoughts are rushing through my mind when I realize there is bright light all around Momma's head. It is as if she has a halo above her head. 'What is that behind her head?' I wonder. Leaning forward and straining to see, I stare in wonder at what looks like little people jumping up behind and around Momma. They are looking at her as though they are straining to see Momma's face!

ANGEL IN DISGUISE

This would be the last time I would personally witness these glorious events. James remains in the room until just before Aunt Pauline arrives from the airport but he never indicates that he saw anything other than Mother's body. I haven't left the room since ten minutes after five. I don't want to miss the powerful and moving events taking place.

(Carol)

I look over at James, his hands cover his face and his elbows are on the bed; he is crying openly. I see movement and realize suddenly, that I'm seeing a head with long, wavy, dark hair. It's flowing in a soft, wavy motion with greyish light trailing behind it and it is moving towards James. "James, it's coming towards you. It's going between your arms." Then it shot into his chest.

"I hope it is with me," he sobbed.

(Pat)

I'm looking at Mamma's spirit right above her body. The SPIRIT shoots upward from Mamma's head and comes, real fast, right to me and stops at the foot of the bed within two feet of me. I could reach out and touch it. It is a complete square. It is just as white as it could be and there is a face inside the square with hair that is really wavy. The eyes, nose, and mouth are black. It's mouth is opening and closing as if talking to me. I can't believe what I'm seeing. A square with a face inside it. I feel the fullness of a complete being before me and my head and heart swim with the wonder of it all. Its eyes look into my eyes and, I feel, into my heart as well. It looks so at peace with itself.

I wanted to talk directly to it, saying, "Hi, how are you?" But I didn't. As fast as it traveled to the foot of the bed, it returns, in a flash, back into Mamma.

Mother is getting worse. Her breathing is very shallow and weak. Mother is going . . .

James is getting all excited, saying, "Hold on Mom. Aunt Pauline is coming." He turns to me and says, "I'm going outside to wait for Aunt Pauline." We know that she is en route from the airport.

(Pat)

It's about ten thirty p.m. and Mary Joe is sitting to the left of Mamma, Carol on the right and I'm at the foot of the bed. The space directly in front of me is misty looking, but the rest of the room sparkles with the brightness of the white light that has appeared. Mary Joe and Carol are both en-circled from head to toe with the bright light. My eyes catch a movement behind Mary Joe. I look.

"Ohhh, they are coming for Mamma. I think it's almost time," I say.

"Why?" replies Mary Joe.

"There are two figures draped in white behind you. Way taller than you. They're behind you, Mary Joe, and back there it is as golden as golden can be."

"I want to see," I cry as I jump from my chair and rush to stand next to Pat. I focus on the area behind the chair I had just been sitting in. I gaze into a radiant glow of white light and a brilliant band of gold want-ing so badly to see what Pat is talking about, but I never see the two figures. I stand there for a few more minutes knowing that Mother is nearing the end and I want to be beside her when she dies. I return to my chair.

(Pat)
Mary Joe gets up from her chair. It's like a spotlight shining directly down on the chair where she sat only a moment before. Even though the color of the chair is black, everything in that area is a bright white. When she goes back to sit down she is immediately framed in the bright light from head to foot.

My eyes are on the two figures. 'Who are they?' is the thought racing through my mind as I begin to see a third figure appearing behind Mary Joe. It is taller than the other two. I'm beside myself with emotion and I scream, "I'm telling you, they're coming. They're here to get Mamma!! There is a third figure behind you Mary Joe."

(Mary Joe)
I look at Pat and shout, "They can't have her." I throw my right arm back behind the chair. What is wrong with my arm? I jerk my arm back and look at it. It feels like my arm had entered an electrical field, leaving a tingling sensation with the hair on my arm standing on end.

(Pat)
My concentration shifts to the right of Mamma. I watch Carol, holding onto Mamma's right arm, begin to bring her hand up and then back onto

Mamma. I watch her hand go from Mamma up through the SPIRIT and back through the spirit and onto Mamma's arm.

(Carol)
I grab for Mothers arm yelling, "Just wait Momma, Aunt Pauline is coming. Just, hang in there." I begin to bring my hands up from Momma's arm and return them in a rapid motion. I look down as I reach for her arm. There is a fog-like, gray mist just above Momma and my hands disappear into it as my hands come to rest on Momma's arm. I release my hold and my hands reappear through the mist. There are my hands!! Each time I reach down to hold onto Mother, my hands disappear into the gray mist. There's Momma's arm; I hold it, then bring my hands up and out of the mist again.

A car pulls up outside.

(Pat)
My eyes are fixed on what is going on in the foreground. Instead of bright light, a gray haze fills the area before my eyes. There is movement over Mamma. No sooner do I see the movement, I see the SPIRIT rising up. This time, it is not a face in a square, this is my mamma. The body is young but there is no doubt, I know it's Mamma. She is wearing a long, flowing white garment. What's that on her sides? I look closely and think, 'WINGS.' No, it must be the pillow but it can't be the pillow because I see the pillow through her SPIRIT. And then I see the WINGS.

"She has WINGS!! She has WINGS!! She is beautiful . . . beautiful . . . beautiful." Tears are streaming down my face.

(Mary Joe)
WINGS? Pat said WINGS!! I slide out of the chair to the floor, onto my knees, my arms out-stretched, crying loudly, "Mother has WINGS?" Pat is nodding her head yes.

"My mother has WINGS!!" I cry. There is no holding back my emotions as I realize that Mother is on her way home. From my eyes flow tears of sadness, joy, grief, anger, happiness, love, and praise. My MOTHER is going home in glory!!

(Pat)
I follow the SPIRIT with loving and tear-filled eyes as it glides toward me. The very essence of me takes in this beautiful SPIRIT, my mamma. She is young, her hair dark, long and wavy. Her garment is misty white, long and flows freely as she heads my way. Extending upward and outward past her sides are WINGS of an utmost brilliance. The sparkling silver WINGS continue just past her waist. Her eyes. I see my Mamma's beautiful eyes but she doesn't acknowledge my presence.

She is so close I could reach out and take her in my arms, but it's not my arms that will hold her tonight. She will be in the arms of her Lord. This is no longer her home. Her home is just a step away. She turns toward the three figures, draped in white, waiting for her. Oh, God, what a breathtaking sight. The glowing WINGS are open and full at her back, her hair, swept back and resting at the nape of her neck. She is pure perfection. This was my mamma. No . . . THIS IS MY MAMMA!!

I feel someone rush by me heading toward the bed. 'Not the bed! The SPIRIT . . . ,' I start to cry out, but instead, stop myself. It is Aunt Pauline who has jumped on the bed with Mother. "Mary Alice, Mary Alice, I'm here."

The minute she jumps on the bed, the spirit is gone, everything disappears. All I see is Aunt Pauline holding Mamma.

Mother's eyes open with a blank look and no response, but Aunt Pauline talks away as if Mother understands what she is saying.

Mother is not yet free and will be not be with her Lord this night. But wonderful things are still to happen, validating this glorious and majestic five and one-half hours. This is Heaven at work, preparing to receive one of its own. We have a little more time to prepare this wonderful and glorified soul to take her journey into eternity.

ANGEL IN DISGUISE

Thirteen

Pat and I left the room and went out into the hallway. I grabbed Pat by the arm, "Oh, Pat, did she have gold WINGS? Were they down to the floor?"

"No, but she had the most beautiful silver WINGS and they went down to her waist."

We ran out onto the front porch. I fell to my knees crying, tears rolling freely, falling to the floor. I was holding on to Pat's waist with my hands. "Oh, Pat, tell me, tell me once more how she looked? Tell me again about her WINGS?" Questions, one after the other, flowed from my mouth, not giving Pat time to respond.

Then she started talking. "She was beautiful!! She was beautiful!! She was young, Mary Joe, and so beautiful." Pat's eyes were filled with tears as she continued. "Her hair was dark, long and wavy. When she turned towards the three figures, I could see that her hair was swept back, laying at the nape of her neck. Her WINGS were down to her waist." As she was describing this, her hands made a circular motion from her shoulders to her waist.

"They were beautiful, shiny silver WINGS."

"Pat, you saw Mother on her way. Mother was on her way!!"

All the time Pat was talking her eyes were looking upward, toward the Heaven from which these grand events had come from. "I don't know what happened to her SPIRIT, Mary Joe. When Aunt Pauline jumped on the bed the spirit disappeared. I hope the spirit wasn't hurt. We've got to find it."

"Don't worry Pat, her spirit will remain until her body dies. It is still with Mother."

"Oh, Mary Joe it was so beautiful. She was so beautiful and those WINGS, so shiny."

I stood up, looked into Pat's eyes and we hugged. We held each other closely and cried softly, both of us realizing that what we had seen was truly a heavenly gift.

These magnificent events, to which I was so privileged to be a witness, are now embedded deeply in my brain. I have the pleasure of seeing these scenes over and over again, and will have this pleasure from now on for the rest of my life.

Pat and I went back into Mother's room. Aunt Pauline was lying there cradling Mother in her arms. "Let's sing," she said.

James, Pat, Carol and I stood around the bed and the five of us, each crying, sang, 'Rock of Ages', 'In the Garden','The Lord's Prayer', and 'Amazing Grace.'

Afterwards, Pat, Carol and I left the room so Aunt Pauline could be with Mother for a while. James stayed in the room with both of them.

Fourteen

When Pat, Carol and I got into the living room we started to explain to each other what we had seen.

Carol said, "I saw little people behind Momma's head. They were jumping and peeking over the top of her pillow as if trying to see her face."

"Well, that's not what I was seeing," said Pat.

"I'll tell you what we should do. Let's go into separate rooms and draw what we saw. Now don't try to be an artist, which none of us are, and then we'll come back and compare our drawings," I suggested.

Five minutes later the three of us sat down in the dining room and together we placed our drawings on the table.

I looked at Pat's paper. There was a square with a face in it. I jumped from my chair and yelled, "I saw that face. I saw it two times. Once, when it went behind you and then appeared in front of your chest. And the second time, when it left the bed and traveled up James' arm and stopped at his heart.

Pat sat there with her mouth open looking at my paper and was pointing with her finger to the face in a square that I had drawn. She was trying to talk at the same time I was talking. "Look, look at this! This right here is what I saw!"

Then Pat pointed to some of her drawings. "See, this is the misty haze I saw over Mamma. And this was when you got up from the chair and came down to the foot of the bed after I told you there were two figures behind you. It was like a spotlight shining down on that chair. I mean a spotlight!!"

I started to explain about my drawing of the bed, "All behind the bed was the whitest white I had ever seen and there were gold streaks behind and over the bed. There were nine times I couldn't see Mother because of all this activity going on above her; there were streaks and rays of gold and crystal clear light shooting in all directions. Between the rays were round objects like the top of people's heads. There was white light completely around Pat who was sitting next to the bed."

"I saw bright, white light but most of the bed was surrounded by silver and gray-like lights. There was white and gold light behind Mamma. And there was white light around her head," Pat said. "Also, see this chair. Behind it were the three figures that I saw coming for Mamma. This one is Mamma, leaving. See her WINGS. Oh, she was beautiful."

"Look here, Pat!" Carol interrupted. She pointed to one of her drawings. "It was like something attached to Momma's side." Pat and I looked at the drawing. The three of us looked at each other. No mistaking it, Carol had seen the 'WINGS' from a side view. Carol was excited. "Here, these are like the little people I saw behind Momma's head. They were jumping and peeking over the top of the pillow as if to see Momma's face. There was this big halo behind Momma." One of her drawings had a haze over Mother's body. Just like Pat's.

Pat continued, "When I first started seeing something it was like little balls of light, like a flash it appeared and was gone as fast." Pat then pointed to the drawing of a face. "I could see this face located above Mamma's; I could also see through it, to Mamma. The shaded area was like a shadow on the face. I knew without a doubt that it was the face of Mamma's spirit.

We had not, up to this point, described to one another what we had seen and since we had referred to 'it' mostly as 'The SPIRIT' or 'IT' during the five and one half hours, the drawings we produced let each of us know that we had indeed had similar experiences.

We returned to Mother's room and even though I knew Mother probably didn't know what I was saying, I told her, "I love you, Mother." I then left the room to sleep on a pallet in the living room. Before falling off to sleep I thought back to those five and one-half hours and I knew that my life would be forever changed. The events that took place, the wonderful things I saw, and what my sisters told me they saw, would have to be shared with all peoples of this planet. Through help and guidance from the Higher Being I knew I would not fail!

Later Pat told me that she, Aunt Pauline and James sat and talked for a while in Mother's room. Then Pat said, "I'm going to sit here with Mamma tonight."

"No need for you to stay up Pat.Why don't you lay down. Aunt Pauline and I are going to sit here with Mom," said James.

"Okay, but if y'all want to go to sleep, wake me up," Pat told them before she drifted off to sleep.

Mary Joe's drawings of her experiences with Mother's spirit.

Drawn around 12MN. Jan.18, 1990

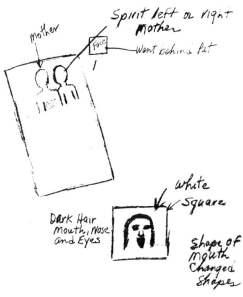

Mother

Spirit left or right
Mother

Face

Went behind Pat

/

White
Square

Dark Hair
Mouth, Nose
and Eyes

Shape of
mouth
changed
Shapes

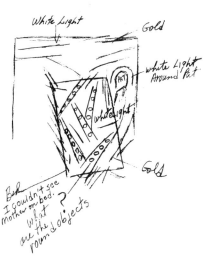

White Light

Gold

White Light
Around Pat

PAT

White Light

Gold

Bed
I couldn't see
Mother on bed.
What?
are the objects
round

121

ANGEL IN DISGUISE

Pat's drawings of her experiences with
Mother's spirit.

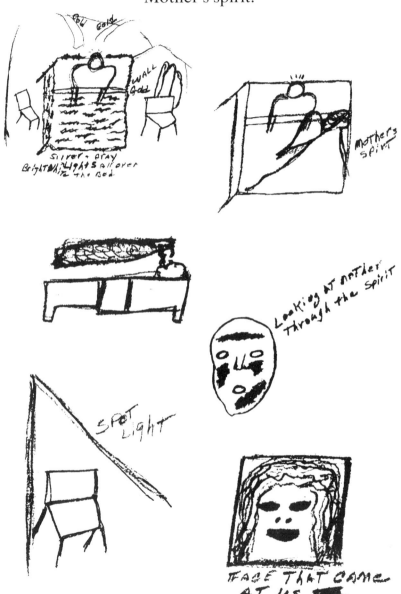

Carol's drawings of her experiences with Mother's spirit.

James crying with spirit coming up his arm.

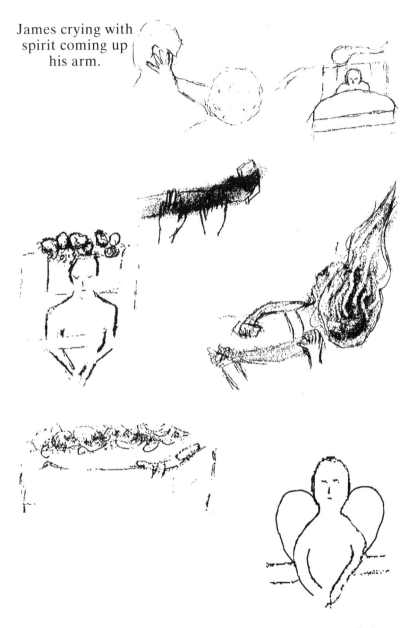

ANGEL IN DISGUISE

Fifteen

My eyes opened and I was struck with the fear that something was wrong in Mother's bedroom. I had gone to sleep on a pallet in the living room at about twelve-thirty. Aunt Pauline had wanted to stay with Mother that night so I agreed to sleep in another room. It was getting pretty crowded in that little room with all the family wanting to be near Mother. I jumped up, ran down the hall and into her room and found everyone asleep. Aunt Pauline was bent over with her head resting on the bed. Mother lay there with her eyes open. I walked over to the bed and looked down at her. Her breathing was shallow, very slow and she was gulping for air. She was still stiff and rigid and her whole body was extremely cold. Her head was tilted toward me.

"My precious baby. You were all alone, but I'm here now," I said. I climbed onto the bed and Mother coughed. The odor coming from her mouth was putrid and made me feel like I would vomit, but I took her in my arms and settled down next to her. I carefully cradled her head onto my chest and ran my hand lovingly over every inch of her face and rested it on her arm. "I love you, Mother," I said over and over again.

It felt wonderful to lay there beside Mother and be close. I held her tiny, stiff and cold body next to me. I had the fleeting thought of placing Mother's face against my chest, stopping her breathing and it would all be over for this loving soul. In my heart I wanted to help end her suffering, but my head knew I couldn't. 'How much more time will I have left with her?' I knew it wouldn't be long.

I thought about those wonderful five and one-half hours that we had experienced earlier that night. "Mother, it was beautiful to be able to see where you're going. What a wonderful gift you and God gave to Pat, Carol and me tonight. I do know now, without a doubt, there is LIFE after DEATH. I've known this through my faith, but now I have seen!! It's so hard to let you pass on but I know that for your SPIRIT to leave we must let your body go. Oh, Mother, how easy it is to say those words but so hard to abide by them. I know it's selfish for me to want to keep you here. It will be so lonesome without you. I can't even imagine my life going on without you, but I know God will comfort me through this crisis. But, oh Mother, I want you to stay!! I will miss you so. I don't know whether you know what I'm saying to you, but if not, maybe you know that someone who loves you more than life itself is holding you oh, so close." I cried softly until I fell back to sleep.

Throughout the night I awoke several times

and on one of those occasions I could feel heat being generated by Mother's body. She was no longer stiff, her body now very limber. She was no longer gulping for air, her breath deep and even. I could not believe it!! What was keeping her alive? Was it the love and energy from us, her children. I drifted back off to sleep.

I felt a hand on my arm and opened my eyes to see Pat leaning over Mother, her face close to mine. "Mary Joe, how is Mamma's heart?"

"I don't know, Pat, but look at her breathing. Her respiration is better than mine. Feel her, she's warm and limber."

Pat felt her. "Mamma, what are you holding on for?" Pat said.

I told Pat about my thoughts of holding Mother's face to my chest and ending it for her.

"Oh, Mary Joe, you remember when the nurse was telling us about how to give the Roxanall under Mamma's tongue to keep her relaxed. And I asked her, 'What if we give too much?' She said that Mamma would just go to sleep and not wake up. She would just die. Well, there was a time when Mamma was real restless and it was my turn to give the Roxanall. I went over and opened the bottle and filled the whole dropper with medicine. I thought this would put Mamma to sleep and she probably wouldn't wake up again. But I couldn't do it, Mary Joe. I squirted it all out except for the 1\2 cc like the nurse had told us. It's so hard to see her in pain like this. She was always such an active person. But I still want her as long as I can have her. Oh, Mary Joe, we've got to let Mamma go. What is holding her here?"

"I don't know, Pat. I don't know. But I guess, maybe WE ARE."

Within the hour the rest of the family was awake. Mother hadn't eaten or drank anything for a week. Would this be her last day of life? At that point, I don't believe any of us would have attempted to make any prediction.

The nurse aide was due to come at ten o'clock to bathe Mother but the time came and went and no nurse aide. Carol phoned the Allcare Agency as I got into the shower to freshen up.

Pat came into the bathroom. "The nurse aide is sick and won't be coming. The agency said they might be able to find someone else." There was a pause from Pat, then she continued, "Mary Joe, why don't we bathe Mamma ourselves?"

"That's fine with me," I said.

By the time I got through bathing and getting dressed, Pat had a pan of warm water, lotion soap, a towel and wash cloth on the table by Mother's bed.

We began bathing Mother, starting with her face and head and working down to her legs and feet. We washed every inch of her body. Aunt Pauline was getting the bed linens together while we finished Mother's bath.

"Mother loves Oil of Olay," I told Pat. "Let's put it on her body." We were both crying as we lovingly rubbed her with the lotion. "It's like they prepared the Lord after he was crucified," I said aloud and looked up at Pat. She looked into my eyes and sobbed openly. No other words needed to be spoken.

When we had finished I ran my hands across Mother's face, arms, chest, legs and feet. Her body felt like velvet, it was so smooth and warm. We changed her bed and placed her on her right side. What an experience we'd had; the preparation of Mother to leave this world. One of the many treasured moments of the week for me to remember about her.

Mother had lost so much weight that her mouth was drawn inward, her lips almost touching the back of her throat. It was as if something had sucked everything out of her. No matter, though, this was still my beautiful MOTHER.

Pat said, "Mary Joe, I'm so worried about what happened to Mamma's spirit last night. I haven't seen it since Aunt Pauline jumped on the bed with Mamma."

"Don't worry, Pat. The spirit will be with Mother until she draws in her last breath of life. It must remain until the body lets 'IT' go."

"I hope so. I just hope that the spirit wasn't hurt or frightened when Aunt Pauline ran into the room, jumped on the bed and put her arms around Mamma. I know that Mamma wouldn't be here now if that hadn't happened. Oh, Mary Joe, it was so beautiful to see Mamma's spirit leaving. And then the little spirit didn't get to go." Pat began to cry.

"I know, Pat, but maybe it was meant for Aunt Pauline to be able to talk, one more time, with Mother. You know, sometimes there is unfinished business to take care of even if there is only one person doing the talking. But look at it this way, if it had finished last night we wouldn't have had this glorious time bathing and preparing Mother for her journey to meet her GOD."

Later in the afternoon I was standing at the foot of Mother's bed and noticed a movement above her body. Then the spirit moved to the left of Mother's body. The SPIRIT is here!! I didn't say anything to anyone. I wanted to just let the spirit lie there in peace above Mother. The spirit was waiting for its time to go. It was waiting for Mother to pass on. We had received our gift last night: that of watching her spirit for five and one-half hours. Mother needed to receive her gift, hopefully, today, that of Eternal Life!!

Sixteen

So much had gone on throughout the week in that room, but life was also going on outside the room. James had come to Carol's house on Monday morning, January 15, without bringing any additional clothes. He also needed to go by his office, which was located between Carol's house and his own and check to see if he needed to take care of any business before the weekend. James left about three o'clock.

Natalie had used my car to go to the bank on Wednesday to take care of a deposit for me and had locked the keys, the only set, in my car. It was Friday and I needed to get the car out of the bank's parking lot. I called American Association of Retired Persons, of which I'm a member, and made arrangements for someone to meet me at six o'clock in the parking lot to help me get into the car.

I called Pat into Mother's room. "Pat, I'm going to leave sometime between five and five-thirty to go by my house and then go meet the person that can get the keys out of my locked car. I hate having to leave. I've been here since Sunday night so if Mother dies while I'm gone, it wasn't meant for me to be by her side when she leaves. Pat, if it really looks like she's going, please tell her that

I love her. And Pat, don't worry about the spirit. I saw it over Mother earlier today."

"You did? Why didn't you tell me at the time?"

"Because it's time to let Mother go. And knowing the experience we had last night I knew it was enough to fill our hearts for the rest of our lives."

Natalie came by to pick me up to go get the keys. Before leaving I went to Mother and bent over and gave her a kiss. "I love you, Mother." Her eyes were closed and I don't know whether she heard me or not, but that's okay.

We went by my house and picked up a few personal items, then left to get my car. We got to the parking lot at six o'clock. We got out of her car since the weather was quite nice for this time of the year. We stood there in the parking lot talking when Natalie suddenly looked up into the sky toward the West.

She said, "Would you look at that sunset." The reflection of the sun hitting the clouds fashioned a sky that was blood red, creating the most striking sunset that I have ever seen. We stood there looking up for the longest time until the AARP representative arrived and opened up the car.

Since I was about one mile from the home of my son Jim, I decided to go by there before I went back to Carol's. I knew my grandchildren, four year old Shannon and thirteen year old Christopher, were visiting their dad and it had been several months since I last saw them. Also, it had been three weeks since I had seen my ten year old granddaughter Starr who lived with her dad. I walked to the door and knocked. Jim slowly opened the door, looked into my eyes and said, "Grandma, is gone. Sue [Carol's daughter] just called me, hoping you might be over here." I fell into Jim's arms and cried. Shannon and Starr came over to me and both said, "I'm so sorry you're sad," and then left the room, only to return within minutes. They handed me a folded piece of paper, and on the outside they had addressed it: to Meme, to Grama, from Shannon and Starr. I unfolded the paper and on the inside they had taken crayons and put streaks of seven different colors on the page with the words, 'I am sorry Meme.' The colors tore at my heart. These precious children had put the colors of the rainbow on that page. The rainbow, a sign of the covenant that God made with man.

I met Natalie back at my house and we drove together to Carol's. "You know, Natalie, I want to live as long as I can, but what I saw last night in Mother's room left me knowing without a doubt where I'm going when I die; Mother will be waiting there for me when I leave this life to begin another, and so will all my relatives and friends that have gone before me.

I walked into the house and went directly to Mother's room. Pat and Carol were there. They had Mother lying on her back, her eyes and mouth closed. The bedding was straightened around her and they had placed her arms down at her sides. Mother looked so nice, as if she was asleep. I went to the bed and laid my body across her's and cried. "Mother, oh Mother, I love you so. Why, why did this have to happen?" Pat and Carol quietly left the room. "I hate that Dr. Matson. I blame him for letting the cancer grow for nine months. Now I don't have a mamma." I stayed in the room with Mother for a while longer then I left the bedroom and went into the living room where Pat, Carol and James were sitting.

Carol said the nurse had been called and when we were ready just let her know and she would come over. It was close to eight o'clock and we had been able to have time alone with Mother, so Carol made the phone call to the nurse. She lived in the general area of Mesquite, where Carol's home was located, so she was there within minutes. Even though Mother had passed away nearly two hours earlier, the nurse had to pronounce her dead at eight-twenty when she listened for, and did not find, a heart beat. She talked to Carol and Pat about what time Mother actually died, and they said Mother had died at about six-thirty-eight; about the time I was looking up into the sky at the blood red sunset.

The nurse then picked up the bottle of Roxanall and had Carol go with her into the bathroom. She poured the liquid into the sink, turned on the water and washed it down the drain. It was time to phone the funeral home to come and get Mother's body.

Two men arrived from the funeral home and the nurse gave them all the information they needed before they could remove Mother's body from the house. Then they brought in a stretcher and went down the hallway. We stood there watching them. One of the men said, "I don't believe the stretcher will fit into the bedroom. We need to carry her out here. I'll go in and wrap Mrs. Davidson in the sheet."

James was standing near the stretcher and he said, "You can go in and put the sheet around Mother but her children will carry her out of that room." The man from the funeral home went in and came out saying that she was ready.

We walked into the bedroom; it would be the last time that we would go into that room and see Mother lying in the bed. Her face was left uncovered. I went to the head of the bed with James next to me, then Carol and Pat. We were all crying uncontrollably, tears streaming down my face and at times, I couldn't see Mother since my eyes were so filled with tears. I placed my hands and arms under Mother's head and neck. James put his hands under her shoulders and back, Carol's hands were placed gently under her buttocks and Pat took her legs and feet. When we were ready we lifted her lovingly, and with reverence, up off the bed. Then we carried Mother out and layed her on the stretcher. We had brought Mother home from the hospital and placed her in that room where she died with dignity, on January 19, 1990 at six-thirty-eight and we, her children, brought her out of that room with dignity.

As the men pushed the stretcher into the living room we asked them to give us a few more minutes with Mother. We stood around Mother and cried openly, our hearts breaking over the loss of this wonderful woman. I could never have asked for a better mother. I had the BEST. We were still crying as we quoted Psalms 23.1-6:

The Lord is my shepherd; I shall not want.
He maketh me to lie down in green pastures: he leadeth

me beside the still waters.

He restoreth my soul: he leadeth me in paths of righteousness for his name's sake.

Yea, though I walk through the valley of the shadow of death, I will fear no evil: for thou art with me; thy rod and thy staff, they comfort me.

Thou preparest a table before me in the presence of mine enemies: thou anointest my head with oil; my cup runneth over.

Surely goodness and mercy shall follow me all the days of my life; and I will dwell in the house of the Lord for ever.

And I thought, 'How true, how true. For I know without any reservation that Mother is, right now, dwelling with her LORD.'

The men from the funeral home then took Mother's body out of the house at about ten o'clock. The house suddenly felt empty.

Dwight wanted to know if we wanted to eat. He had cooked dinner earlier but didn't think we would want to eat until the people from the funeral home came for Mother. I put the first bite into my mouth but found I couldn't swallow. Pat was sitting beside me. She jumped up from the couch and ran down the hall crying and screaming, "Mamma! Mamma!" with Jack, her husband, in close pursuit. "Jack, I don't know what I'll do without my mamma."

I told Carol I was going to go on home. It would be the first time I had been home for the night in five days. It felt good to lie down on my own bed, but memories of the things I did with Mother rushed through my mind and it was impossible to go to sleep. I cried softly until I fell asleep.

Seventeen

Saturday morning I left home to meet James, Pat and Carol at Restland Memorial Park to make the funeral arrangements. Our appointment was for one o'clock. After being ushered into the office, we found the Director with Mother's file on the desk in front on him. James and I sat across from him and Carol and Pat sat on a couch positioned near the desk.

We knew Mother had bought two grave plots and a funeral program back in 1971. The Director let us know that the last payment of twenty-two dollars was due. I couldn't believe it, THE LAST PAYMENT. She really had it all mapped out! We were told the only remaining cost would be the flowers, newspaper notice, concrete vault, opening and closing of the grave, and the grave-site name marker.

Other than these items, this caring woman had once again showed the loving concern she had for us, her children, by making all these critical decisions nineteen years ago. She had picked all the colors, from the casket to the interior of it and had written in the plan that she wanted her eye glasses in her hands, as if she had just taken them off for a moment to rest her eyes and then fallen to sleep.

The Director asked us, "What do you want us to do with her jewelry, her necklace?"

"She didn't have a necklace on," I said.

"This cross, she had with her." And he pulled out of the file, a Xerox copy of the cross. We all laughed and cried at the same time. We now knew that the cross was somewhere on Mother when she left Carol's house going to the funeral home and we knew she had not gone alone. Throughout the whole week that we had been with Mother, each one of us had placed or pushed the cross onto her chest as she lay in the bed. Our fingerprints on the cross had accompanied her. We asked the Director where they had found it. He wasn't able to give us an answer. I know that we couldn't find the cross on Friday afternoon when we discovered it missing. We had looked on the bed, under the sheets and over every inch of Mother's body. And I mean every inch. We couldn't find it. Now, there it was! It had been on Mother, but where? Then we knew, it was meant for us to make this trip with Mother, if not physically, then through our love in making sure the cross was always lying on Mother's chest near her heart.

The Director told us Mother would be ready for us to view around five o'clock. It was almost four, so we decided to go over to the floral shop. We ordered red roses for the family casket spray and an arrangement of pink roses and baby's breath to be wrapped around the top and bottom of a picture of Mother that was going to be at the head of her casket. The picture was of her when she was twenty

The cross and form from the funeral parlor.

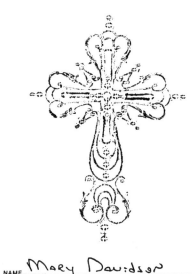

NAME Mary Davidson

CASE NUMBER _____

NAME Mary Davidson

CASE NUMBER

F.D.	RECEIVED BY	RECEPTIONIST	DATE
DELIVERED	RECEPTIONIST	INITIAL	PICKED UP

ARTICLES CHECKED IN:

Cross

_____

_____

_____

_____

_____

_____

_____

Signature of person receiving valuables

Received by:_____Relationship_____

Address_____

City & State_____

ANGEL IN DISGUISE

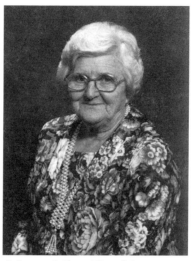

Mary Alice Davidson

DAVIDSON

Mary Alice, age 77, died January 19, 1990 at the home of her daughter. Born August 13, 1912 in London, AR. She moved to Dallas in 1956 and lived for many years in the Mesquite area. She was a former resident of Lakeland Manor in Dallas where she lived 10 years prior to her illness. Beloved mother of Mary Joe Risher, Mesquite, James David Davidson, Irving, Patricia Ann Bolton of Texas City, Carol Jean Myrdahl, Mesquite; sons-in-law, Dwight Myrdahl & Jack C. Bolton, Sr.; grand-children, Deanna & (Kenny) Ginger, Sue & (John); great-grandchildren, Justin, Nicholas & Daniel, Christopher, Starr & Shannon; Shaun, Brittany & Tiffany; Erin; brothers, Cecil (Christell) & Joe Jr. (Lorene) Petray, Malvern, AR; sisters, Aline Baker, Dardanelle, AR, Pauline Reddell, W. Richland, WA; Joan Ballard, Arkadelphia, AR; sister-in-law, Alice Petray, Malvern, AR; host of nieces, nephews & friends. Services 2:00 P.M. Monday, RESTLAND MEMORIAL CHAPEL. Interment Restland Memorial Park. Pallbearers will be the grandchildren: James & Richard Risher, Bill & Jennifer Myrdahl, Britt Davidson & Brian Bolton.

RESTLAND

Greenville Ave. at Restland Rd.

236-7111

years old. We also went ahead and ordered the flowers for her from the grandchildren and great-grandchildren.

The time had come for us to go into the viewing room. We walked in and there was my precious MOTHER.

James, Pat, Carol and I walked over to the casket and looked down at Mother. When the mortician prepares a body, he or she is not able to make the person exactly like you remember them. Close but not exact. I thought they did a good job on Mother but Carol had wanted less filling in the jaws and mouth as Mother never was one to wear her false teeth. Pat and James never commented one way or the other. Mother didn't wear lipstick so they removed it from her lips and applied a very soft gloss to them.

Mother looked like she was sleeping. She had her eye glasses lying on her chest and was holding the little white Bible and cross that she had held close to herself for the last two months of her life. The turban Pat had given to her for Christmas was on her head and made her look noble. The pink bed jacket and pajamas matched perfectly with the pink lining of the casket. She had made a great choice in color, one which made her look so natural.

Carol asked if they still lit candles near the casket. The Director informed her it was usually done if the person was Catholic, and she replied that Dad had had them positioned at the head and foot of his casket and he wasn't Catholic. She explained the reason she wanted to know was that she burns those candles for a few minutes every Christmas in memory of Dad and had hoped to have the candles from Mother's funeral.

At this point I noticed that the crystal I had taped to the little heart pillow that Natalie had given to Mother for Christmas was missing. I had given Mother the crystal and had placed it in her pillow-case ever since she started her treatments. I asked where the crystal was. The Director looked in the casket around where the little pillow was placed but was unable to find it. He left to see if it was among the other personal things of Mother's. Pat said, "Mary Joe, I believe I have a crystal here in my purse." She looked, then emptied the contents out onto the table. There it was. She handed it to me and as I was taping it to the pillow, the Director came in carrying a box with Mother's items in it. Sure enough, there was the crystal. I picked it up out of the box and taped it to the pillow and handed Pat's crystal back to her. She said, "Can't my crystal go with Mother, too?"

"Sure it can, Pat." Pat handed it to me and I walked over and laid it beside Mother's right leg. We both carried crystals in the belief that crystals would add positive energy to our lives.

The Director told us that the room where Mother was lying is actually two rooms, but since they did not need the extra room they had opened up the folding doors to allow us to have more space. There were several tables with lamps, a couple of chairs and a small couch. This was quite comfortable for those wanting to visit Mother.

Satisfied with the arrangements, we all went back to Carol's house. Liz and Marie were there when we arrived. Marie said she wanted to talk with us privately so we went into the bedroom where we had taken care of Mother for those three months. Pat and I sat on the couch while Carol sat on the bed. Marie stood in front of us. "I went to bed last night, and of course my thoughts were of you girls and the loss of your mother. I had a dream and I wanted to tell you what I dreamed.

"There were three women in a hallway and a room with blue carpeting. The three women were crying and saying, 'We don't have our crystal, we can't get in.' One of the women came to me, and Carol, I knew it was you because the woman wore her hair like you. She said, 'I don't have the crystal lantern. I don't have the crystal lantern.' I turned to this woman and gave her a crystal lantern but the other two women kept saying, 'But we don't have our crystal, we can't get in.' I woke up and on the night stand was my crystal lantern like the one I saw in my dream, so I knew that I must give it to you Carol. Also, I knew that Mary Joe and Pat needed to have their crystal."

She gave me a cut lead crystal egg and Pat, cut lead crystal coasters. When Marie was through I said, "Now let me tell you what happened today." I told her what Carol had said to the Director about the candles that had been placed at the head and foot of Dad's casket, and that she was hoping to get the candles that would burn near Mother's casket. I then told her about the lost crystal from the pillow and about Pat giving me her's and having found the crystal, but Pat wanted her crystal to go with Mother, too, so I placed it by Mother's right leg. I looked at Marie and said, "By the way, in the room where Mother's casket is, the carpet is BLUE."

The five of us remained in the room talking. Then I asked Pat to tell me what happened after I had left on Friday to go get the car.

"After you left, Carol and I were in the room talking. It began to get dark and I left the couch, walked over to the foot of the bed and looked at Mamma's body, wondering what had happened to the spirit. I know you told me you had seen it, but I had to try and satisfy myself that the spirit was still there. All of the sudden, I saw the spirit. At about that time, Carol turned on a small lamp on the dresser. As soon as she had turned it on, she said, 'No, I'm not going to leave it on because the neighbors can see in,' and she turned the lamp off. There the SPIRIT was, right there, just a little bit above Mother, lying on its side. I just went, 'Aaah!!' I looked at Carol and walked out of the room with Carol asking, 'Did you see it? Did you see it?'

" 'Yes,' I replied.

" 'I did too,' echoed Carol. At about that time, the phone rang and I went to answer it. It was James David wanting to know how Mamma was and I told him that her breathing was shallow, real shallow and he said that he was on his way back over. While I was talking, another call came through. You know, Carol has call waiting, so I switched over. It was the nurse, so I gave the phone to Carol. Just as Carol started talking to her, Sue, who had been in Mamma's room for several minutes, stepped out of the room and said, 'Grandma's eyes are open.' I hurried back into the bedroom and yelled for Carol to get back to Mamma's room. She ran in still talking to the nurse on the phone. She told the nurse, 'Momma is dying now. She's breathing like a little fish out of water.' But Mamma's eyes were not wide open like she was scared or anything. You know, her eyes were glassy, set and staring but there was a soft look in her eyes. Aunt Pauline wanted to get to Mamma so bad, but Carol and I said, 'Let her go! Let her go, Aunt Pauline!'

"We were crying out that we loved her. Then I said, 'Mamma I love you . . . Mary Joe loves you ... Carol loves you ... James loves you... Richard, Jimmy, Billy, Sue, Jennifer, Britt, Ginger, Deanna, Brian, Erin and all your great-grandchildren love you.'

'MOTHER.
HAVE A WONDERFUL JOURNEY!'

"She took about three or four breaths and then died. Carol picked up the stethoscope and walked over to Mamma and listened for a heartbeat. She looked at me, shook her head and said, *'she's gone.'* We cried.

"We straightened Mamma up in bed. Carol had told the nurse that we would call her when we were ready. You know, we just wanted more time with her, we didn't want to give her up right then. We knew that you and James would need your time with Mamma.

"While we sat in the bedroom waiting for you and James to come back, Carol told me what she had seen right after she had turned off the light in Mamma's room. 'Pat, there were heads of people all over the bed. They were at Momma's chest, arms, stomach, knees and hips. They were everywhere on the bed. They were waiting for Mom, Pat!!'

"I heard a car drive up so I left the bedroom and went into the living room. James came running into the house and looked at Sue saying, 'Grandma? Grandma?' Then he looked at me, 'Mamma? Mamma?' I told him that she was gone and he ran down the hall and into her room. 'I wanted to be here. I wanted to be here. I was here for five days. I was here for five days.' I told him that if it had been meant for him to be here he would have. James was devastated."

I looked at Pat after she got through telling me all that had happened while I was gone. "Well, Pat, Mother was right when she told you two years ago that you would be with her when she died. You and Carol were the ones chosen to send Mother off on her next life's journey. I feel bad about not being here when Mother passed on, but I believe what is meant to be, will be. I hope James understands that, too. It was not meant for either of us to be here at that time."

Eighteen

I left Carol's house about nine o'clock. When I got home I told Natalie all we had done that day and that the picture of Mother was going to be placed at the head of the casket.

She said, "It's nice to have the picture of your Mother when she was young. Since her friends at the high-rise only knew her in her senior years, wouldn't it be nice to have your Mother's life, in pictures, displayed in the viewing room."

"That would be great, Natalie. I have a lot of pictures of Mother taken over the years." I went into my closet and pulled out albums and boxes of pictures.

Now would come the job of choosing the pictures to be used. Natalie had an assortment of portfolio's to put the pictures into once I picked those to be displayed. I was sad about Mother's death, but there was an air of excitement in putting together the story of Mother's life in pictures. I found pictures of her from when she was in her twenties until now. Natalie offered to help me since it was so late. She mentioned it would be nice to create an every-ten-year account of Mother's life in pictures. I even had a newspaper article written back in 1972 about our trip to Hawaii with a picture of Mother and Don Ho taken, when we attended the Don Ho Luau. Natalie took all the pictures and put together the display. We had worked through most of the night to get it ready to take and set up in the viewing room. I appreciated what Natalie had suggested and that she had helped put together this picture tribute to Mother. Tired, I fell quickly to sleep.

Sunday morning I awoke around eight o'clock. I wanted to get to the funeral home and get the pictures arranged before noon. I took a shower, dressed and decided I should try to eat breakfast before I left, but food was not something I had been able to deal with since Mother's last week of life and her death. Maybe it was because I knew Mother hadn't eaten anything that week. It was like I shouldn't eat either and found it was hard for me to swallow the food once in my mouth.

We arrived at the funeral home and since we had use of the extra room, there was plenty of space to put the pictures on display. I've never attended a funeral where there was a pictorial story about the deceased. It was different and it was certainly a wonderful tribute to this remarkable woman.

I stayed in the room with Mother so I could see and talk to her friends when they came to pay their last respects. I could tell it was hard on these women when they viewed Mother's body. Pat or Carol were in and out of the room throughout the day and when no one else was in the room, it gave me time to just be with MOTHER.

Early in the afternoon, my son, Jim arrived with his family. Two of my grandchildren went over to Mother's casket to look at her. I started to pick up Shannon, my four year old granddaughter and take her over to see her Grandma Davidson, as she called Mother, but Jim said not to. I didn't say anything, but felt that we all need to experience closure.

I left the funeral home about five o'clock and went by Carol's for dinner. She had told James and I to come by her house since her neighbors had brought food over during the day for the family. At a time like this, most people can depend on their neighbors. I have never been able to thank them personally, but if they read this book about this wonderful woman, I want to say, "Thank you for what you did to make things easier for the Mary Alice Davidson family, on January 20-22, 1990."

Pat, Jack and their son, Brian David, came over to my house on Sunday evening to spend the night. Mother's brothers and sisters began to arrive from Arkansas on Sunday. Several hotel rooms had been reserved for them in a hotel up the street from Carol's house with several family members staying at Carol's.

I didn't sleep most of the night. I cried a lot knowing that when the sun went down tomorrow it would all be over and life would go on. But it would go on without me being able to see my Mother ever again.

ANGEL IN DISGUISE

Nineteen

Monday morning arrived and I awoke and went into the kitchen to start breakfast. I moved routinely, not making conversation with anyone. Today would be the last time I would have to touch or kiss the physical body of my beloved MOTHER and when I thought about this, I would get choked up.

I went into the pantry to get a box of cereal for Brian and directly in front of me, on a shelf, was a bag of black-eyed peas. I chuckled as I picked up the bag and brought it back into the kitchen. I put the peas in a pan of water and let them cook while I got ready to go to Carol's. Arrangements had been made for the funeral home limousine to pick the four of us up at her house. Finally, we were ready to leave and I went into the kitchen, poured the cooked peas into a jar and capped it. Now I was ready to go, jar and all.

At one o'clock the limousine arrived and we were on our way to Restland's Wildwood Chapel where the service was to be held.

I went into the chapel and found flowers every-where throughout the room and all around the casket. I took the jar of black-eyed peas and placed it on one of the pedestals behind a floral arrangement.

Later, just before the two o'clock service began, I was talking to Carol and several of Mother's friends from the Senior Citizen high-rise when Sue came up to us and remarked, "Did any of you see that jar of peas on the pedestal at the foot of Grandma's casket? I wonder who would do that?"

"I did," I answered.

"You did?" was Sue's response.

"Yes. Many times I've heard Mother say to people when they were talking about death or funerals, 'Rather than sending me flowers, you can bring me a bowl of black-eyed peas.' The response would be, 'black-eyed peas! You can't eat those peas.' And Mother's answer would always be the same, 'I can eat those peas as well as I can smell those flowers.'"

We all broke into subdued laughter.

The chaplain from the hospice program was asked if she would officiate at Mother's funeral. Carol had made arrangements months ago with her friend, Father Luke* and he had agreed, but death is not scheduled by appointment and when Mother died he was on vacation. The hospice chaplain said she would be happy to perform the service.

The pallbearers would be five of Mother's grandsons; Jim, Richard, Britt, Bill, Brian and one of her granddaughters, Jennifer. She had held, loved and baby-sat each of those six grandchildren when they were young. There they sat, all grown adults now and it was right that they should be the ones to carry her those last few feet to the grave-site.

The chaplain was talking about who Mary Alice Davidson was and those whose lives she had touched, family and friends. She continued, "One of Mary Alice's daughters, Patricia, has written two poems in tribute to her mother. Patricia read these poems to her mother several years ago. A privilege not all of us will have, that of knowing what will be read at our funeral."

TRIBUTE TO OUR MOTHER
from her children
written by Patricia Bolton

God came and took you from us.
He holds your loving hands.
He wants to show you his world now,
A world that is so grand.

God must have said;
Mary come go with me,
I'll show you wonders you've never seen.

My Garden is a Paradise.
My Streams are crystal clear.
There will be more love in Heaven,
Now that you are here.

I will walk beside you,
Every step of the way.
We will walk and talk together,
For MARY this is your day

So take my hand,
It is time for us to go.
I will take care of you now,
FOR I LOVE YOU SO.

ANGEL IN DISGUISE

The song 'In The Garden' was sung at the end of the poem. The selections, 'In The Garden,' 'Precious Memories,' 'Old Rugged Cross,' 'Rock Of Ages,' and 'Amazing Grace,' were songs Mother had loved and indicated she would like to have played or sung at her funeral.

The chaplain continued with the tribute in poem.

> *MOTHER it is time for us to say good-bye,*
> *It is time to let you go.*
> *Our grief we must try to endure*
> *For we also loved you so.*
>
> *Words cannot express,*
> *The way we feel today.*
> *Our hearts feel like they are broken,*
> *Our MOTHER has gone away.*
>
> *MOTHER was a warm, a tender, a loving*
>   *and caring person.*
> *Helping others was her goal.*
> *All her friends will miss her,*
> *For they also loved her so.*
>
> *You are away,*
> *Yet ever so near,*
> *Your voice, your smile will be everywhere,*
> *For us just a memory away.*
>
> *Although you will no longer be seen,*
> *By family or by friends,*
> *You will live, because you were dearly loved,*
> *AND LOVE CAN NEVER END.*

The words were still pounding within my heart as 'Precious Memories' was being sung. 'Oh, how strong are those memories I hold so dear of my mother. There will be no future to remember, only memories and they flood my head with happiness and joy. I will be able to recall these treasured memories at any time for the rest of my life. Oh, those precious memories.'

With the service now over, it was time to go to the grave-site...but, one last look at Mother. Mother! Mother! My legs could hardly hold me up to walk to the casket. I know James, Pat and Carol were having their own emotions to deal with as we all made our final trip to say good-bye. I stood before the casket, looked down, reached out and touched Mother's hands and then her face. Then I bent over and kissed her lips. My last contact with this WOMAN who had given me LIFE.

We got into the family limousine and watched Mother's grandchildren carry her casket and place it in the hearse. Now we would follow this remarkable woman in her lifetime, for the last time!! As the limousine we were in came to a stop, the casket was being lifted out of the hearse by her grandchildren. I watched my own two sons, Jim and Richard, and my heart cried for them. My thoughts went back to the many times Mother had been around them and had wanted them to spend the weekends with her. The memories of the four years that we had lived with Mother after their father and I were divorced. I can see Mother now, carrying three-year-old Richard over to the baby-sitter as we got ready to leave for work in the mornings. In later years, during holidays, Richard would call and tell Mother, "Grandma, I want to put my order in for two pecan pies and two pumpkin pies." She was a fantastic cook and we all knew it.

She was with me at the hospital when Jim was born and she was with me when I brought him home. Jim was her first grandchild and both Mother and Dad spent a lot of time with him during his childhood. Then my eyes went to Jennifer. When we were talking about who would be the pallbearers and named the grandsons, we came up with five. Someone mentioned another male member of the family, but he was not a grandchild. I said, "Why don't we ask Jennifer if she would like to be a pallbearer? After all, who says a pallbearer has to be a male. Mother carried her around when she was a baby just like she did the boys." Mother loved her grandchildren and they loved and respected her, the Matriarch.

We got out and walked to the grave-site. The chaplain conducted a short service and it was time for us to go. GO!! LEAVE!! It was so hard to turn and walk away from Mother but we had to. The casket had to be lowered and covered and the funeral home personnel wouldn't do that while we were still there.

The limousine took us back to Carol's house and as we walked into the house we found it full of people who had known Mother. Carol and Mother's neighbors had brought food and placed it in the dining room, kitchen and den. There was enough food to feed the whole residential block. It all looked good but, right then, I didn't think I could eat anything.

Mother's brothers, sister-in-laws, sister and nephew needed to get started on their trip back to Arkansas so we all went out into the front yard to say our good-byes. Natalie asked me if I wanted her to take a picture of the whole family before they left and I told everyone it was picture taking time. We all grouped together and the picture was taken. Uncle Cecil said as he got into the car, "You all keep in touch with us."

After they left, Natalie turned to me and said she wanted to take a picture of the four of us. As we positioned ourselves for the picture, my thoughts went back to times in the past when the family had gotten together and we always had our picture taken before we left Mother and Dad's house to go home. Before Dad died there were six of us in a picture. Before Mother died there were five us.

With our arms around each other's backs, we stood together and the picture was taken of the four of us.

Afterwards, we stood in the front yard talking to each other and I turned and looked at James David, Patricia Ann and Carol Jean. As I looked into the faces of my siblings, I wondered, 'Who will be left for the picture of three?' And at this thought, MY HEART CRIED.

ANGEL IN DISGUISE

Why

While I was writing this book, I found I was going through the grieving process, which made me realize that I had not completed my grieving as I thought I had.

One day I had just finished writing about the last night of Mother's life on this earth. I was crying, feeling physically, emotionally and mentally drained.

When I'd finished writing for the day, I would read it to Pat or Natalie for feedback. There were times I was crying so hard, the words were a blur through my tears.

"Why? Why me? Why us? Why did I have to write this book about what my sisters and I saw?" I said.

"Why not you?" was Natalie's response.

I replied, "Why not one of the great spiritual leaders"

"Why do you think something like what you saw would only be for a spiritual leader? Maybe, Mary Joe, you were open to what you were privileged to see, and it was known by the Higher Being that you would tell and share what you saw."

I accepted that as being as good an answer as any to my 'WHY' question.

Several weeks later I was in Ariel Bookstore, in Vancouver, B.C. I saw a book about women of the Bible. I walked over and picked up the book. The page it opened to had to do with the ascension of

ANGEL IN DISGUISE

Jesus. It was to WOMEN that He first appeared.

After getting home, I went to the little Wildwood Chapel. I often visited the chapel to sit and meditate before writing. I picked up the Bible and turned the pages to the ascension of Jesus in each of the books of Matthew, Mark, Luke and John.

I had asked the questions: Why me? Why us? Why am I to write this book?

The answer was before my eyes in Luke 24.1-11. The women took spices, which they had prepared, to the sepulcher. And they entered in and found not the body of the Lord Jesus. There were two men in shining garments and they said unto the women, quoting from this passage. "Why seek the living among the dead?" The women remembered Jesus' words and returned to tell the apostles that Jesus had arisen, but those words seemed to them an idle tale, and they did not believe the women.

The women JESUS appeared to were: Mary Magdelene, Jo'Anna, Mary the mother of James and other women. The question was answered:

MARY JOE   (MARY) M.   (JO)Anna
Patricia ANN   Jo(ANN)a

My mother MARY was the mother of JAMES
I am also MARY, the mother of a JAMES

I was in shock; the answer couldn't have been any clearer. It had been written almost two thousand years ago by the disciples that this would happen; that we WOMEN would see and tell about this glorious and spectacular transition from this life into the next.

I will bear witness for the rest of my life, to what my sisters and I saw that night of January 18, 1990, the night my mother was preparing to take that step into her next life journey. I'm comforted, in that I know I will see her again.

All questions are ANSWERED.

MarJoe Davidson